Case Studies Through the Healthcare Continuum

A Workbook for the Occupational Therapy Student

Case Studies Through the Healthcare Continuum

A Workbook for the Occupational Therapy Student

Patricia Halloran, MBA, OTR/L
Center for Technical Education, Quincy, MA

Nancy A. Lowenstein, MS, OTR, BCN
Boston University, Boston, MA

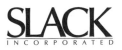

6900 Grove Road, Thorofare, NJ 08086

Published by: SLACK Incorporated
6900 Grove Road
Thorofare, NJ 08086 USA
Telephone: 856-848-1000
Fax: 856-853-5991
www.slackbooks.com

Contact SLACK Incorporated for more information about other books in this field or about the availability of our books from distributors outside the United States.

Library of Congress Cataloging-in-Publication Data

Halloran, Patricia, 1967–
Case studies through the health care continuum : a workbook for the occupational therapy student / Patricia Halloran, Nancy Lowenstein
        p. cm.
ISBN 1-55642-405-1 (alk. paper)
1. Occupational therapy—Case studies. I. Lowenstein, Nancy, 1953– II. Title.
[DNLM: 1. Occupational Therapy—Case Report. WB 55 H192c 2000]
RM735.45 .H354 2000
615.80515—dc21
00-026537

Printed in the United States of America.

Last digit is print number: 10 9 8 7 6 5 4 3 2

DEDICATION

To my family, all the students who have inspired me to be a better instructor, and all the patients who have taught me so much.

Nancy Lowenstein

To my parents, Daniel and Muriel Halloran.

Patricia Halloran

Contents

ACKNOWLEDGMENTS

The idea for this book was born out of my desire as an instructor to bring the clinical reasoning process to my students. All the textbooks that I used had students develop treatment plans, but no other critical thinking skills were asked for. Thus, a student could become very good at writing the initial treatment plan, but not know what to do in treatment if things didn't go as they planned. So the idea for a book of cases and questions was planted and shared with my colleague Trisha Halloran.

I would like to thank my co-author, Trisha, for being the driving force behind getting this book written. Without her "let's do it" attitude, I would not have had the drive to do this alone. I would also like to thank my colleagues who read cases and provided constructive feedback, specifically Cathie Marqusee, MS, OTR, and Jody Kaufman-Smith, OTR. Special thanks to the staff at SLACK Incorporated for guiding me through this process.

Most importantly, thanks to my family for putting up with my countless hours at the computer.

Nancy Lowenstein

A special thank you to Marcy Harris, OTR/L, CHT for offering her expertise in upper extremity orthopedics; to Frank and Chris Chenette for their computer/graphics assistance; to Tom Chenette for his creative ideas; and to the Rehab II students at QHS/CTE for posing for the illustrations. I would also like to thank Janet Meade for her illustrations and Frank Perrault for his cover drawing. Most importantly, my gratitude to all the patients who have taught **me** about rehabilitation.

Patricia Halloran

Part I

Introduction

This book was born out of our frustration as instructors that most case studies in current texts asked only for treatment plans and goals. The real-life situations that we saw as practicing therapists were not well represented in these case scenarios. Students were not asked to think about the steps after the treatment plan was completed and actual treatment was begun. This is, we feel, where a truly flexible and adaptable student does well on fieldwork. It is this ability to realize that working with real clients requires flexibility, adaptability, and a sense of humor. Often our best attempts to predict outcomes fail because of circumstances that we didn't anticipate during our initial evaluation; maybe because of family issues, health issues, or client-centered issues. Therefore, our goals for this textbook are to assist students in learning that there can be many possible choices in the clinical decision-making process, and that these different choices can lead to many equally successful outcomes. Mental flexibility and thinking on your feet are important clinical skills to cultivate, and students must learn that there are very few "black and white" decisions in clinical practice. By developing these skills, one can cross the bridge between a well-educated student and a competent clinical practitioner.

Each case in this book provides information about the patient's physical, emotional, and interpersonal skills. This information acts as a guideline for the student as they progress through the questions, starting with goals and treatment planning and ending with discharge planning. Each response to a question creates another clinical pathway for the student to examine; each response will affect the answer to the next question(s). The various pathways that develop allow students to compare their work and see that many different responses can be appropriate for the same case.

This book is not intended to teach theories and constructs for clinical reasoning. Furthermore, it is not meant to teach occupational therapy students or occupational therapy assistant students how to evaluate. The students are expected to use the information provided by the case histories and occupational therapy evaluations. Students should be able to explain the rationale for their answers to each question, as this book is intended to provide a vehicle to put theories and clinical reasoning into practice before reaching the clinical fieldwork stage of training. Doing so will help students to reason out how to deal with the many different scenarios that they may encounter during their clinical placements. While one can never be prepared for everything that may happen during fieldwork, we feel these cases offer a very realistic picture of each clinical setting and raise the very difficult questions that students will be asked.

Suggestions for Use of This Book

We see this text as a workbook to encourage students' clinical reasoning skills. This book can be used in many different ways and is only limited by the skill and imagination of the instructor. We have purposely not used a specific frame of reference for this book for several reasons. This allows each college or technical program to fit the book to their specific frames of reference and enables instructors to use various frames of reference with different cases. In a few of the psychiatric cases, however, the Model of Human Occupation and Allen's Level of Cognitive Disabilities are mentioned. These questions can be easily rephrased with another frame of reference or even deleted if the instructor wishes to do so.

In many of the cases, we do not provide specific details. This is to encourage students to look up information and find resources outside of their classroom texts. Again, this is a skill that students will need in clinical practice and as they further their clinical education. We encourage instructors to add or delete information in order to enhance or refocus a case or to fit with the academic level and knowledge base of their class. Instructors may have students complete cases or certain questions several times simply by adding or omitting details. This would allow them to compare how different clinical pathways, treatment and outcomes can be when only one detail changes.

Additionally, instructors may assign one half of the class with a case with information deleted/changed and the other half with information remaining unchanged. This will generate interesting discussions, comparison, and learning. In addition, we encourage instructors to bring their own clinical experiences and theoretical orientation to the discussions of the cases.

For class use, cases can be assigned as group or individual projects, as work to be done during lab, or as assignments outside of class. In addition, the cases can be used to initiate discussions about different aspects of patient treatment. Although we have grouped the cases by settings, they do not need to be followed in this order. Cases may be designed by diagnosis, age, or even by specific section such as Self-Care/Work/Leisure or Psychosocial. Students may use the Notes section to jot down ideas and questions, as well as answers.

We feel this textbook can be used in many different classes and even used during the same semester by different classes. In examining input from various program instructors, students can see how information is integrated from different course areas to provide holistic occupational therapy treatment. This is also beneficial for the program because it enhances the curriculum and provides a connection that is often missing between classes. Cases may even be completed again by the same group of students as they progress through their coursework. This gives them the opportunity to compare how they would react to a situation as, for example, a third year student and again as a fourth year student. Allowing students to reflect on changes they might make with more knowledge and experience gives them the opportunity to grow as clinicians. Both professional and technical programs can use this text. A good use would be to have classes in both a professional and technical program work on the same case and to explore how the OTR/COTA relationship works.

Most importantly, all students want to become competent therapists and are often hungry for the **right** answers. All instructors have witnessed students who have gotten stuck when presented with information that does not have clear answers. As practicing therapists, we know the importance of realizing that rehabilitation is an evolving process. The therapeutic relationship and the occupational therapy treatment plan changes frequently during that process. By understanding this, students can practice how to make the changes positive instead of trying to block them.

Again, students need to be reminded that there will be many different answers to the same questions. They may find different answers among classmates and even among different instructors in the same program. They can then evaluate, with the help of their instructors, which responses they think will work best for the patient and for themselves as therapists. By doing so, it will also foster the development of the skills of therapeutic use of self.

We encourage instructors to be creative in the ways they use this workbook, to use it as a tool to encourage students to think "out of the box," and to help students understand that cookie cutter treatments are not possible in occupational therapy.

Part II

Acute Care Hospital

Chapter 1

Adam:
Myocardial Infarct,
Coronary Artery
Disease

Adam is a 56-year-old Caucasian man brought to the emergency room by his wife after complaining of chest pain, indigestion, and heartburn that had been going on for several hours. He was admitted to the coronary care unit (CCU) with a diagnosis of myocardial infarction (MI) and coronary artery disease. Adam's MI is of moderate nature with damage to the heart evident on EKG. Additional diagnoses include gastric ulcers and tendonitis of the elbow. Adam has not had a physical in years and has no documented history of heart disease. Adam is 5'8" and weighs 200 pounds. Prior to his MI, he was independent in all his daily life functions. He is a highly successful executive for a technology firm. He has been married for 31 years and has two sons; one son is away at college, and the second is a junior in high school. His wife, Janine, works full-time as a chief financial officer for a chain of retail stores.

Adam and his family live in a large, two-story colonial home in the suburbs with four bedrooms and two full baths upstairs, and a half bath and living areas on the first floor. He can enter the house from the garage up five steps. Once inside, he must manage a long flight of stairs to get to the second story.

Adam loves to golf and sail and he takes his family on two vacations a year to pursue these activities. He wakes early and comes home late. He drinks large amounts of coffee and smokes two packs of cigarettes a day. His father died at the age of 62 of a heart attack. Adam is a driven man who expects everyone around him to excel and to extend themselves to the fullest. He works an average of 70 hours a week. He enjoys his lifestyle and his roles as worker and father the most, although he spends little time with his family. He is a confident man and states he doesn't let difficult situations get to him. Adam denies that stress is a factor in his life and says he thrives on challenges. He is planning to return home immediately following his hospitalization and to return to work quickly.

He is being seen by OT and PT immediately after his discharge from the CCU onto the cardiac floor of the hospital.

Occupational Therapy Evaluation

Adam is evaluated 1 week after his MI. He is evaluated on the coronary care floor, not the CCU. Adam presents with no deficits in cognition, perception, sensation, vision, or hearing.

He has AROM WNL, with good coordination; he is left-handed. His strength is not tested due to his cardiac status, but appears functional for current tasks. He has significant deficits in endurance, with his sitting tolerance out of bed only 5 minutes. He can transfer from the bed to the chair and from sit to stand with contact guard. Supine to sit requires minimum assistance and his bed mobility is independent using bed rails. He can ambulate without devices and walks short distances (bed to bathroom).

He has some ecchymosis on his hands from the intravenous lines.

Currently, he is dependent for his ADLs and IADLs. He is quite fearful and anxious since his MI. He feels he has lost control of his life. He does not want to die and has been thinking a lot of his father's early death from heart disease. He did not like the environment of the CCU and did not sleep well while there.

He is cooperative and wishes to actively participate in his rehab program and to return home, and expects to be back at work within 2 weeks—he says he doesn't trust the work to get done without him there. He has already started to contact the office by phone. Adam's goals are to return home and to work as soon as possible. His expected length of stay is 2 weeks.

QUESTIONS

Goals/Treatment Plan

1. Please write a problem list for Adam of the issues that need to be addressed during his acute care hospital stay.

2. Based on the goals Adam has expressed, write a list of long- and short-term goals for occupational therapy treatment.

3. Do the goals Adam stated coincide with the OT goals? Why or why not?

4. What functional activities will you use to reach these goals?

5. Knowing that Adam's expected length of stay in the acute care hospital is only 2 weeks, what discharge plans would you recommend for Adam at this time? List Adam's strengths.

6. Please write a treatment plan for Adam, include methods and activities (include appropriate metabolic equivalent, [MET] for each activity).

Safety/Precautions

7. What are the signs and symptoms of cardiac stress that you must watch for during your treatment sessions with Adam?

8. What vital signs should you monitor before, during, and after each treatment session, and how do you monitor them? What are the normal parameters for these vital signs?

9. What safety issues should you address with Adam regarding his return home?

Self-Care/Work/Leisure

10. Please describe the patient education program for Adam concerning his ADL routine.

11. What ADL activities are appropriate for Adam to participate in during his acute care hospital stay?

12. Briefly describe a treatment session to address Adam's ADL deficits.

13. Would you teach Adam breathing techniques to use during his ADL routine? If so, what breathing techniques would you teach him, and how would you recommend he incorporate these into his ADL routine?

14. How would you address Adam's work role? What do you see as important issues for Adam to understand in this area?

15. How would you address Adam's leisure activities?

NOTES

Equipment/Adaptations

16. What, if any, adaptive equipment might you recommend for Adam to use during his ADL routine? To his work routine?

17. What type of adaptations would you recommend Adam make to his home? Would these adaptations be permanent or temporary?

Neuromusculoskeletal

18. What type of UE activities would you recommend during his acute care hospital stay?

19. What are the maximum METs that Adam should achieve during his acute care hospital stay?

20. What type of patient education would you provide Adam regarding his exercise program?

Cognition/Perception

21. Stress is an important risk factor in MI. How do you think occupational therapy should address this in treatment with Adam?

Psychosocial

22. Please identify any issues you feel affect Adam's psychological health.

23. Why are these issues as important to address in his treatment as his physical issues are?

23a. Would you consider referring Adam to another discipline for psychosocial issues? Which one(s)?

Patient/Family Education

24. What would you identify as being important for Adam to change in his lifestyle, and how would you educate him in these areas?

24a. How would you educate Adam about the role of stress and myocardial infarction?

Situations

25. Adam's wife asks to speak to you privately. She tells you that she is afraid to let Adam return to work, golf, or sailing, and doesn't know how to get him to give up his leisure interests. How do you handle this situation?

26. Adam's wife also says that she is afraid of resuming a sex life with her husband. How do you handle this situation?

26a. Do you feel it is the role of OT to deal with a client's sexuality? If not, who should? How comfortable are you in dealing with this area?

27. You enter Adam's room to start treatment and find him on the phone with his office. He is quite agitated and angry. When he gets off the phone you take his blood pressure and find that it is 200/120. How do you handle this situation?

28. Adam tells you that he wants to start a daily exercise routine and to purchase some equipment for his home. What equipment do you suggest that he buy and why?

NOTES

29. You recommend that Adam return to the hospital as an outpatient and participate in the stress management classes and cardiac rehab program that are offered. He says that he thrives on the intensity and doesn't find it stressful. How do you respond to this?

Discharge Planning

30. How would you address Adam's insistence that he return to work after his hospital stay and not go to the hospital's cardiac rehab program?

31. Adam's acute care hospital stay is brief. Given that Adam insists on going home and returning to work instead of attending a cardiac rehab program, what would your discharge instructions include?

NOTES

Chapter 2

Beth:
Radical Right Mastectomy,
Right Upper Extremity Lymphedema

Beth is a 43-year-old Asian-American female with a diagnosis of breast cancer resulting in a radical right mastectomy and subsequent right upper extremity lymphedema. For this reason, she has opted to have the right breast and surrounding tissue removed. Beth's mother and aunt both died from breast cancer and she feels strongly that she does not want to take any chances. In addition to the surgery, Beth has been receiving radiation.

Beth is married and has two sons, ages 15 and 12. She and her husband own and operate a catering business together. Her husband, Brett, manages the finances, advertising, and booking customers. Beth creates the menu and the presentation. They have two part-time employees and had wanted to expand the business before Beth got the news about her breast cancer from her physician. Beth is also active in her sons' school and sports activities. She is a "sports mom" for Jason, her older son, and takes Jarred, her younger son, to karate and swimming each week. Beth had no functional limitations before her surgery. Her busy work and family life left her little time for leisure activities. "Cooking was my hobby, now it is my life!" she says. She does, however, enjoy evening walks with her husband and family camping trips.

Occupational Therapy Evaluation

Beth's surgery was performed on a Tuesday and she was seen by occupational therapy on Thursday morning. Her Wednesday occupational therapy appointment was cancelled because she had so many visitors earlier in the day. She refused an evaluation that afternoon. However, Beth was seen by physical therapy on Wednesday. She had gotten out of bed and walked a short distance (about 50 feet). She will be discharged home on Friday.

Upon evaluation, Beth has no cognitive, perceptual, visual, hearing, or sensory deficits. She has normal ROM in all limbs except her right UE. She is right-hand dominant. Her AROM in her right shoulder is as follows: flexion: 30°; extension: 0°; abduction: 15°; adduction: 0°; internal and external rotation: not tested related to pain. Beth has full extension in her elbow and 110° flexion in her elbow. She has normal wrist and hand motions. Strength was not tested in her right UE.

Beth complains of pain and tenderness in her incision area and distal to the procedure. She has ecchymosis in the surrounding area and 1 to $1\frac{1}{2}$" edema surrounding her shoulder joint to bicipital groove area. She has 1" lymphedema from the midhumerus to the midforearm area. The edema is more prevalent on the anterior portion of the limb than the posterior. Beth wears a swath sling for the right arm.

Beth transfers herself in and out of bed independently and ambulates independently without a device. Beth requires minimum assistance for bathing her left arm due to limited ROM in her right arm. She also needs minimum assistance to dress her upper body. Beth has been wearing only a johnnie, underpants, and slippers for comfort and ease. Beth requires moderate assistance to don and doff her sling.

Beth requires assistance for all two-handed activities, such as cutting food, opening a door while carrying items, and many household activities. Beth complains of fatigue but is insistent on going home tomorrow. She agrees to meet with occupational therapy later today and before she leaves on Friday afternoon. She says her goals are to "go home and get my life back to normal."

QUESTIONS

Goals/Treatment Plan

1. Devise a problem list for Beth.

2. Write a list of Beth's strengths.

3. What specific goals would you and Beth set for your two occupational therapy treatment sessions?

4. Write out a specific treatment plan for each of your two sessions with Beth.

Safety/Precautions

5. To what precautions must Beth adhere, given her recent surgery?

6. Why are such precautions necessary?

7. How could occupational therapy help Beth to adhere to these precautions?

Self-Care/Work/Leisure

8. Explain how you could instruct Beth to adapt her bathing and dressing routines to foster greater independence.

9. Name five work-related tasks that Beth would be unable to do at this time.

10. State how adaptations could be made to the tasks so that less assistance would be required.

Equipment/Adaptations

11. What type of adaptive equipment might benefit Beth? Explain why.

Neuromusculoskeletal

12. What occupational therapy treatments would you recommend for the lymphedema?

13. How could these treatments be carried out given that Beth is leaving the hospital tomorrow?

14. What type of ROM activity would you recommend for Beth's right UE?

15. Write out your recommendations and restrictions.

Psychosocial

16. What type of psychological impact do you imagine the surgery has had on Beth?

17. What do you think some of her fears may be regarding her diagnosis and postop status?

18. What type of impact do you think Beth's surgery and diagnosis might have on her husband? On her sons?

19. What are some community supports available to Beth to cope with her diagnosis? Find three, two of which should be in your geographical area.

NOTES

Patient/Family Education

20. What specific education would occupational therapy need to provide for Beth's family?

21. What type of education should be provided to Beth and her family by the nursing staff?

Situations

22. Beth asks you how long it will be before she can use her arm normally again. What do you say in response?

23. Beth asks you why her right arm is so swollen. How would you explain it to her?

Discharge Planning

24. What type of occupational therapy would you recommend for Beth after discharge? Explain why.

NOTES

Chapter 3

Craig:
Spinal Cord Injury at C-5, Complete

Craig is a 36-year-old Asian male who fell off a ladder while fixing a sign at the retail store he owns. His employee saw the fall and called 911 after it was clear that Craig could not get up. He was transported to the nearest emergency room where he had an MRI, which determined that he had sustained a complete fracture of the spinal cord at the C-5 level. Craig is in good health and has no known medical conditions. He was placed in the ICU to await surgery for a halo vest. After 2 days, it was felt that Craig was medically stable and surgery was performed to place him in a halo vest. He was transferred out of the ICU onto a medical unit.

Craig is married and has no children; he and his wife were waiting until Craig's store was economically stable. Craig opened his music store, selling CDs, tapes, and DVDs, 18 months ago. Craig has two part-time employees, and he spends about 70 hours a week at the store. His wife, Elaine, works full-time as a receptionist in a doctor's office. They live in a large city in a 5th floor apartment; there is an elevator in the building. Their apartment is a small one-bedroom apartment, with one bathroom and a galley kitchen; the living room doubles as a dining area as well.

Both Craig's and Elaine's families live in nearby communities. Their families are immigrants from Korea; both Craig and Elaine are first-generation Americans. Their families are proud of them and their achievements. Both families are devastated by the news of Craig's accident. Family ties are close and Craig's parents continue to hold beliefs from their Korean culture about family and health. Craig has two sisters. One lives nearby and works full-time, and the other is currently living and working in Korea.

Craig is a quiet, confident man. He is soft-spoken with a wry sense of humor. He has an optimistic outlook on his life. Craig believes that hard work and persistence will lead to success. He is a college graduate. He and his wife have a strong marriage and share the same cultural heritage and beliefs. He is bilingual, speaking both English and Korean fluently. His leisure interests include biking and hiking. Craig worked in retail prior to opening up his own business. He hopes that his business will be able to support his family so that his wife can stop working when they have children.

Occupational Therapy Evaluation

Craig is seen immediately after the halo vest is applied. He demonstrates no deficits in cognition, perception, vision, or hearing. His sensation is absent distal to C-5. In addition, he is dependent for all ADLs, transfers, and mobility.

Craig has flaccid paralysis throughout his UEs and LEs.

Craig had been immobilized on a kinetic bed until his halo vest had been applied, and was able to tolerate supported sitting up for 10 minutes during the evaluation, before he began to complain of feeling nauseous and dizzy. Craig asked to continue the evaluation at another time. During the occupational therapy evaluation, he appeared despondent, angry, and confused. He does not seem to understand what a complete spinal cord injury means and is frustrated that no one will tell him if he will walk or hug his wife again. His goal for therapy is to do what he must to get to the rehabilitation hospital. His expected length of stay is 2 weeks if no medical complications arise.

Questions

Goals/Treatment Plan

1. Given that you were unable to complete the OT evaluation, what additional information would be needed to devise a treatment plan?

2. Given the level of Craig's injury, what muscles would be fully innervated and what muscles would be partially innervated?

3. Given the information in question 2, what motions would Craig have in his upper extremities?

4. How would you assess Craig's upper extremity strength?

5. What role, if any, would the COTA have in this case?

6. How would you educate yourself about cultural factors that may be important for Craig's recovery and your treatment planning?

Safety/Precautions

7. What is the name of the severe medical emergency that can be life-threatening to a spinal cord injury patient? What are its symptoms, and what are the actions you should take if this happens when you are working with Craig?

8. What is orthostatic hypotension? What are its symptoms and what should you do if Craig experiences this while you are working with him? What precautions must be taken with Craig, due to his immobilization in bed?

Self-Care/Work/Leisure

9. What might you address in the area of self-care with Craig during his 2-week stay? Why did you choose this area?

10. Given the level of Craig's injury, do you think he will eventually be able to dress himself? Please explain your answer.

11. Given Craig's business, do you think he can successfully return to his store after rehabilitation? Please give the rationale for your answer.

12. How will you instruct Craig in pressure relief? Why is it important for Craig to learn to do this? What other discipline would be responsible for education in this area?

Equipment/Adaptations

13. What adaptive equipment might you give Craig to start using in the acute care hospital?

14. Write a prescription for a wheelchair for Craig. This should include the type of wheelchair, any customized seating systems, controls, or other features.

NOTES

Neuromusculoskeletal

15. Why does Craig have flaccid paralysis? Is this common in spinal cord injury? Will spasticity develop in his muscles?

16. What treatment techniques would you do with Craig to address his muscle weakness?

17. Please write an exercise program for Craig to perform on his own while in bed.

18. What type of splint would you make for Craig, and what is the goal of wearing the splint? Write out a wearing schedule for Craig's splint. What should staff be educated to look for when taking off his splint?

19. How will occupational therapy assist Craig in developing sitting tolerance? Please explain your treatment techniques.

20. What is the safest method to use in transferring Craig from his bed to his wheelchair? What treatments might OT and PT work on together? How can you document this to be sure there is no duplication of service?

Psychosocial

21. Discuss the stages of psychological adjustment to physical disabilities. What stage do you feel Craig is experiencing?

22. What are some of the common coping mechanisms that individuals use in dealing with traumatic injury? Please comment on the positive or negative impact each may have on recovery.

23. What psychosocial supports are currently available to help Craig deal with his emotional state?

Patient/Family Education

24. The acute care hospital is the first environment where Craig, his wife, and their families will learn about spinal cord injury. What types of information would you give them at this time? Where will you look for information? Can you find any organizations or support groups in your area for spinal cord injuries? Write them here.

25. There are several risks associated with spinal cord injury, and Craig and his wife need to do daily checks for some of these. What are these risks, and how do you educate Craig and his wife about them?

26. Craig's wife wants to be an integral part of his care. What activities can she do for him to help maintain his musculoskeletal integrity?

Situations

27. You are working with Craig and he starts to perspire, complaining of a pounding headache and chills. What does this indicate and what is your response?

28. During treatment sessions, Craig talks constantly about the day that he will walk. It motivates him to do his exercises and gives him hope. How might you handle this?

29. Craig has developed moderate spasticity in his lower extremities and mild spasticity in his upper extremities. He is anxious about this change and thinks this means he is getting worse. How might you explain the presence of spasticity to him? How can spasticity be useful in your treatment program?

NOTES

30. One afternoon you enter Craig's room to find it filled with family members from both sides. They have set up a small shrine and seem to be involved in some sort of religious practice. Your schedule is very tight, and this is the only time you have to see Craig in the afternoon. What do you do?

Discharge Planning

31. Craig has been at the acute care hospital for 2 weeks and is ready for discharge to a rehabilitation facility. Write a discharge summary using the following information: Craig is currently in a wheelchair 2 hours a day; his wheelchair has been ordered. He has had several episodes of orthostatic hypotension and autonomic dysreflexia, and has developed spasticity. Include other information from the case history, family, and psychosocial issues.

NOTES

Chapter 4

Donald:
Traumatic Brain Injury—Ranchos Level II

Donald is a 26-year-old Caucasian male. He is a professional race car driver who suffered a TBI following a spectacular crash at one of his races. He was pulled out of his car unconscious and treated immediately at the track by EMTs who stabilized him enough for transport to the hospital. In the ER, he was given CT scans, x-rays, a tracheotomy, catheter, and IV, and an intracranial pressure monitor was inserted into his brain. He was comatose, and, in addition to his head injury, suffered two fractured ribs, a left fractured humerus and radial/ulnar wrist fracture, and a right fractured femur. He was sent to the intensive care unit (ICU). He had no other significant medical history.

Prior to his accident he functioned independently in all areas of self-care, work, and leisure. Due to his career, he was on the road for 7 months out of the year, traveling to different parts of the country to race. When he was not racing, he stayed at his parents' house in a rural community. Both his parents are living, and his father is still working as a police officer. His mother does not work, but is very involved in her church and helps the elderly congregants with shopping, chores, and visits. Donald has a younger sister, who is married with a 6-month-old child. She lives in a community near her parents. He has an older brother who is also married and lives 1,500 miles away with his wife and four children.

Donald was a friendly and outgoing person. He was very popular on the race car circuit and enjoys a "good time" out with the guys after the races. Donald always loved cars and began working on his father's car when he was 12. He bought his first race car when he was 17 with money he saved from odd jobs and fixing other people's cars on weekends. He played varsity football in high school. He opted to join the race car circuit immediately after high school graduation. He is a confident man and a good race car driver, with a good driving record and a few wins. He is well-respected by his peers on the circuit. Although he likes to drink, he has never driven while under the influence. He is a lady's man and has no desire to settle down in the near future. He loves to dance and his favorite musician is Garth Brooks. He tries to take in a concert whenever he is able. He has a dog, a mutt named Scoundrel, who travels with him in his small motor home.

Because he has no health insurance, his parents want him to stay with them during his recuperation. They say that they can take care of him and are sure the community will support them in their efforts as well. Already, the pastor of his mother's church has put out a request for help from parishioners for when he returns home.

Other team members include the neurologist, ICU nurses, physical therapist, respiratory therapist, and speech therapist. The acute care hospital where Donald was taken has a very good TBI team.

Occupational Therapy Evaluation

Donald was evaluated 1 week post-accident, when he was medically stable but still in the ICU. According to the medical record, Donald sustained a closed head injury with focal damage to the frontolateral cortex. He was comatose when the EMTs arrived at the scene of the accident, and he has not regained full consciousness yet. He is at the Ranchos Los Amigos Level II at the time of the OT evaluation. The nurses have noted some spontaneous eye opening. His left upper extremity and right lower extremity are in casts due to fractures. His digits show 1+ pitting edema, and there are many bruises on his body. He demonstrates moderately increased tone in the right UE and left LE. Passive head movement elicits changes in tone and abnormal reflexes include the ATNR, STNR, TLR, and extensor thrust. He responds to stimuli such as loud noises, pinprick, and quick position changes with a generalized response, going into decerebrate rigidity with the stimulation. Facial grimacing and teeth grinding occur spontaneously. Nursing staff report that he appears more alert and responsive in the morning and again in the early evening. Donald has IVs in his right UE and an intracranial pressure monitor.

QUESTIONS

Goals/Treatment Plan

1. Write a problem list for Donald.

2. What goals would you set for Donald, and how would you include his family in setting the treatment goals?

3. How would you involve his family in helping to reach your treatment goals?

4. How would you educate Donald's parents about the nature of your treatment sessions? How would you anticipate your collaboration with other team members?

Safety/Precautions

5. Given Donald's medical condition, what precautions would you take during your treatment sessions?

6. Given his medical condition, what possible problems might occur during Donald's treatment sessions, and how would you respond to each of these?

7. Write out a list of the possible medical emergencies that Donald may experience at this stage of his recovery.

Equipment/Adaptations

8. What kinds of adaptations will you make to Donald's hospital environment? Why?

9. What might you recommend his family bring in from home to assist with your environmental adaptations?

Neuromusculoskeletal

10. Given the nature of Donald's injuries and his Ranchos level, prioritize his neuromusculoskeletal needs.

11. What do you identify as some of the factors that may interfere with addressing these needs?

12. How will his head positioning influence his tone?

13. How will you position Donald in bed so as to inhibit as much spasticity as possible?

14. What type of devices would you fabricate to deal with Donald's increased tone in his upper and lower extremities? Who would you enlist to assist you in fabricating these devices?

15. How will you know if Donald is responding appropriately to your positioning devices?

16. What type of sensory stimulation will you want to give to Donald and why?

17. How can Donald's family assist you with his sensory treatment?

18. Should Donald's family bring in items from his home to enhance his sensory stimulation? Why or why not? If so, what types of items would you suggest?

19. How will you know if Donald is responding to your sensory treatment?

NOTES

Psychosocial

20. How would you address the psychosocial needs of Donald's family?

Patient/Family Education

21. Identify 2 agencies in your area that provide services and support to individuals and families with TBI.

22. Your hospital asks you to develop a patient/family educational brochure on head injury and the types of care offered at the acute care hospital.

Situations

23. In the middle of a sensory treatment session, in which you are gently stroking and vibrating his left arm, Donald begins to have a seizure. What do you do?

24. Donald has progressed to a Ranchos Level III. What would you now do differently in the areas of sensory stimulation and positioning?

25. Donald has begun to integrate some of the primitive reflexes as well. What types of neuromuscular activities would you use, and what types of movements would you try and encourage?

Discharge Planning

26. By the time of discharge, Donald has been moved out of the ICU and has been upgraded to a Ranchos Level III. How would you explain to his parents what behavior to expect from Donald at this level?

27. Donald's parents really want to care for him at their home, because he does not have insurance to cover any more inpatient stays. What supportive services would you recommend that they obtain, and how would you suggest they obtain them? Do you think it is unethical for Donald to be denied admission to a rehab hospital because he has no health insurance?

28. Write a home program for Donald's parents to follow for Ranchos Levels III and IV.

29. Donald's parents' house is small, and Donald's room is on the second floor. Would you recommend that they set up a bedroom on the first floor or keep it on the second floor? Please explain your answer.

30. Donald's home community is raising money for him to go to a rehabilitation hospital. Write a discharge note so the next OT knows what has transpired during Donald's acute care hospital stay.

NOTES

Chapter 5

Ellen:
Right Total Shoulder Replacement, Rheumatoid Arthritis

Ellen is a 58-year-old Caucasian woman with a diagnosis of right total shoulder replacement. Ellen also has a diagnosis of rheumatoid arthritis. She has a past medical history of bilateral knee replacements and a left hip replacement. Ellen elected to have the surgery when the pain and stiffness in her left shoulder had limited her to a point where she could barely use her right arm. The rheumatoid arthritis had begun affecting her arm about 2 years ago and had gradually progressed to the point where surgery was inevitable. Ellen describes her right arm motion as "minimal" before surgery.

Ellen lives with her son and his family in an apartment adjoining their home in the suburbs. She and her husband have been divorced for many years and Ellen is used to doing everything for herself. She likes being independent and hates "giving in" to the arthritis. She retired from a job with the telephone company 4 years ago. She had worked there for 25 years as a dispatcher.

Ellen reports a gradual increase in difficulty in performing ADLs before the surgery for the last year and a half. She has needed assistance from her daughter-in law to wash and brush her hair, dress her upper extremity, and reach into closets and cabinets. She eats dinner with her son and his family, but eats the other meals in her own apartment. She was independent in cold meal prep prior to surgery. She ambulated with a straight cane because of left lower extremity weakness. She reports this had become difficult since she used the cane on the right side. She reports all daily tasks were difficult and elicited pain throughout the shoulder region. She was unable to continue driving because of her inability to use her right arm to shift gears. Ellen's favorite leisure activities are Bingo and Crossword puzzles. She maintained independence in this area.

Ellen underwent surgery to replace the glenohumeral joint. Her surgery was uncomplicated and she was out of the recovery room to the hospital unit the next day when the occupational and physical therapist greeted her. Ellen wore a swath sling on her right upper extremity. Her doctor had issued total shoulder precautions, which stated she was allowed external rotation to neutral only and no abduction unless the glenohumeral joint was fully internally rotated. Ellen's surgeon had warned her to adhere to the precautions stringently. Ellen had not been so careful in the past and had experienced difficulty after her left hip replacement as a result.

The discharge plan is for Ellen to remain at the acute care hospital for 5 days, then return to her home. She will have her rehabilitation from an occupational therapist from the Visiting Nurse Association. While at the hospital, Ellen is to receive services from OT, PT, nursing, nutrition, and social service.

Occupational Therapy Evaluation

Ellen is pleasant and cooperative during the evaluation. She has no cognitive, perceptual, visual, sensory, or hearing deficits. She reports pain in the right shoulder whenever she moves in bed or ambulates. She is wary about removing the sling for the evaluation, but agrees reluctantly to do so. Her AROM in the right UE is as follows: shoulder flexion: 25°; extension: 15°; internal rotation: 45°; external rotation: 0°; all with pain she rates as 7 to 8 on a scale of 1 to 10. Her elbow and hand are WFL. She does have slight ulnar drift of the 2–5 MCPs on the left hand. Ellen's left UE has AROM as follows: shoulder flexion: 110°; extension: 30°; abduction: 100°; horizontal adduction: 95°; horizontal abduction: 5°; external rotation: 40°; internal rotation: 80°. Her left elbow and hand status is the same as the right side. She is right-hand dominant. Her coordination is impaired due to her limitation of the right shoulder. She exhibits difficulty with manipulation of small objects because of her arthritis and ulnar drift, but is very persistent in performing tasks as asked.

Ellen still has the sutures in her shoulder where the surgery was performed. The area is covered by a dressing that nursing is monitoring regularly. The chart reports that the incision is doing well. Ellen has no edema and reports moving her fingers on the right hand all the time to keep them from feeling stiff.

Ellen requires moderate assistance to move from supine to sit. She transfers with very minimal assistance and ambulates with her straight cane and close contact guard. She is now using the cane in the left hand because of her surgery and has an unusual gait pattern. She reports feeling light-headed and dizzy after getting up to walk or sitting up in bed. Ellen is using a bedside commode for toileting and is calling for assistance with her transfers.

Ellen is able to feed herself, although she reports having very little appetite since the surgery. She requires moderate to maximum assistance with self-care of the upper body. She needs only minimal assistance for the lower body when performed in bed. She performs toilet hygiene independently. She is dependent for all home-management tasks.

Ellen reports familiarity with OT since she had it in the past with her other surgeries. "I know the ropes, unfortunately," she jokes. Her goals for OT are to perform all her self-care tasks independently so she won't need so much help when she returns home. She especially wants to be able to shower herself. "I plan on driving again," she says "but that'll be a while."

QUESTIONS

Goals/Treatment Plan

1. Devise a problem list for Ellen.

2. Write a list of Ellen's strengths.

3. What specific goals would you and Ellen set for occupational therapy given her short length of stay?

4. How might Ellen utilize her strengths to maximize her potential while at the hospital?

5. Write out a specific treatment plan for Ellen including frequency and duration.

Safety/Precautions

6. What are the precautions to which Ellen must adhere?

7. Why are these precautions necessary?

8. How might you explain the adherence to precautions to Ellen so she can better follow them?

9. What functional activities might be unsafe for Ellen to engage in at this time?

10. What might be causing Ellen to feel dizzy when rising for ambulation? Who should you speak to regarding the dizziness? What could be done to reduce it? What activities might cause Ellen to endanger her right shoulder?

Self-Care/Work/Leisure

11. Write out a detailed bathing and dressing treatment session for Ellen. Explain exactly how you would promote independence and what portions of the task you would help her with.

12. Explain how you would address Ellen's dependence in home-management tasks.

Notes

Equipment/Adaptations

13. What type of adaptive equipment might you issue to Ellen to increase her level of independence? Explain why.

14. How might Ellen's hospital environment need to be adapted for greater independence?

Neuromusculoskeletal

15. Write out an exercise protocol for Ellen's right shoulder. Include specific types of exercises. What functional activities will you connect to her exercise program?

16. What could be done within the realm of occupational therapy to treat Ellen's shoulder pain? Would you encourage Ellen to perform exercises for left UE as well? Explain why or why not.

Psychosocial

17. How might Ellen be coping with her fourth joint replacement operation?

18. What social supports does Ellen have to deal with her limitations once she returns home?

19. Why might Ellen have ignored her joint replacement precautions in the past?

Patient/Family Education

20. What type of education will Ellen's family need before she returns home?

21. How can you be sure that she and her family understand the information presented to them?

Situations

22. You walk by Ellen's room and she is leaning out of the bed, trying to pull her commode closer with her cane handle. She is leaning on her affected arm and grimacing in pain. What do you do, and what do you say to her?

23. Ellen would like you to show her how to get out of the bed using the half-bed rails as an assist. Describe the technique and steps you would teach her.

24. Ellen is now able to perform sponge bathing at the sink with minimum assistance for UEs only. She asks if she could try the shower since it's easier and more thorough. What will you need to find out before you begin this type of treatment?

25. How would you set up a shower session for Ellen?

26. Ellen has shown some slight increase in AROM of left shoulder. She asks you how much can she expect to gain before she returns home. What is your reply?

Discharge Planning

27. Ellen is going home late in the afternoon today. She is ambulating independently with her cane and reports no dizziness. You are scheduled to see her once before she leaves. On what might you focus your session?

28. What recommendations will you make for the home OT in your discharge summary?

NOTES

Part III

Rehabilitation Hospital

Chapter 6

Frank:
Right Cerebrovascular Accident,
Left Hemiplegia, Left Neglect

Frank is a 68-year-old Caucasian male with a diagnosis of right cerebral vascular accident (CVA) of the internal carotid artery and left neglect. In addition, he has coronary artery disease and diabetes. Two weeks ago, Frank was brought to the emergency room by his wife complaining of an unbearable headache, with slurred speech, and loss of control on his left side. He was admitted to the acute-care hospital where he was stabilized and an endarterectomy was performed with good results. He was transferred to the rehabilitation hospital for more extensive rehabilitation.

Prior to his CVA, Frank had been a very active man. He recently retired from his job as a postal worker and is looking forward to traveling with his wife and tending to his garden. He is an avid gardener and woodworker and anticipates enjoying his two hobbies more extensively.

Frank has a son who doesn't live nearby, with whom he has a strained relationship. Frank and his wife live in a ranch-style home in a suburban neighborhood. There are 5 steps into the front door, and the garage is not attached to the house. They are friendly with some of their neighbors, but others are new to the neighborhood, and they do not know them well. Frank has always done all the home-maintenance tasks on his home.

Frank has many friends from the post office, and he has maintained his weekly bowling night with them after their retirement. He and his wife have a strong marriage. They are planning on his return home after his discharge from the rehabilitation hospital. He will be seen by occupational therapy, physical therapy, speech therapy, and recreational therapy. He will also be seen by nursing, dietary, and physiatry.

Occupational Therapy Evaluation

Frank has no deficits in his hearing or vision, aside from wearing glasses for distance. Frank does have deficits in perception, with difficulty in figure-ground and spatial relations. He demonstrates right/left confusion and a profound left neglect. Cognitively, Frank shows poor attention span, insight, judgment, and safety awareness. He has difficulty maneuvering around his room and the hospital environment, constantly bumping into things on the left side. Sensation testing finds impaired sensation for light touch and sharp/dull, as well as impaired stereognosis on his affected side.

Frank has no AROM or sensory deficits in his right UE. He is right-handed. He presents with weakness in his left UE and LE, he has poor dynamic sitting and standing balance, and his static standing balance is fair with good static sitting balance. His PROM in his left UE is shoulder flexion to 85°; abduction to 70°; and elbow flexion to 100°. His wrist and hand have PROM WNL, but he has increased tone in his fingers and wrist. He presents with moderate tone throughout the UE, neck, and trunk, and mild tone in his LE. His left UE has AROM as follows: shoulder flexion/extension: 0°–50°; add/abduction: 0°–45°; internal rotation: 0°–5°; external rotation: 0°–15°; elbow flexion/extension: 0°–60°; supination: 0°–15°; pronation: WNL; wrist extension: 0°–10°; wrist flexion 0°–45°; finger flexion: ¼ range. His finger extension is weak. He is unable to release objects. Strength is not tested due to increased tone. Coordination on the left is impaired for both fine and gross motor.

During the ADL evaluation, Frank demonstrates difficulty with right/left discrimination. He has a great deal of difficulty managing his clothing. He is unable to figure out the front from the back or the sleeve hole from the neck hole and needs maximum assistance with all dressing tasks. He appears to have a dressing apraxia. Bathing was completed while sitting at the sink. He neglected his left side totally, didn't attend to objects on the left side of the sink, and needed a great deal of verbal cueing and physical guidance to complete the task.

He ambulates with a hemi walker and minimum assist due to his poor balance. He transfers with minimum assist and moderate verbal cueing due to poor safety awareness. Frank scored a 49 on the Barthel Index.

Frank is very amiable and likes the staff. He teases them and is good at involving humor in interactions with others. He does not understand why he needs so much therapy or why he has to be in the rehabilitation hospital. His wife told him that the doctor said he needed to be here and that is why he stays.

Frank's and his wife's goal is for him to return home and resume his hobbies. He looks forward to picking up his life where it was before it was disrupted by the CVA. Frank's wife is very supportive of these goals and will do whatever it takes to get him home to live life as before.

QUESTIONS

Goals/Treatment Plan

1. Write out a problem list for Frank.

2. What are Frank's strengths and how can these be drawn upon during your treatment planning?

3. What would the long-term goals be, given what you know about what Frank and his wife want? How would you incorporate Frank's wishes into your treatment planning?

4. What are your first set of short-term goals for Frank? What frame(s) of reference will you use and what treatment modalities?

5. If you think that Frank and his wife have unrealistic expectations for his long-term goals for his rehab stay, how will you handle this?

6. What obstacles do you see in Frank reaching his stated goals? What role would a COTA play in Frank's treatment? Be specific in terms of *skills* during evaluation, treatment planning, and treatment sessions.

Safety/Precautions

7. What are the primary safety concerns that should be addressed with Frank?

8. How would you and the team address these concerns?

9. What type of adaptations to the environment or adaptive equipment would you want to use in addressing the safety concerns identified in Question 7?

10. Are there any treatment precautions that need to be taken with Frank?

Self-Care/Work/Leisure

11. What would you identify as Frank's self-care deficits? Why are these obstacles for Frank?

12. How would you set Frank up to bathe at the sink? What kind of physical and verbal cueing do you anticipate he might need and how much?

13. Would you give Frank adaptive equipment for his ADLs? Why or why not? If you would, what kind would you give him?

NOTES

Figure 6-1.

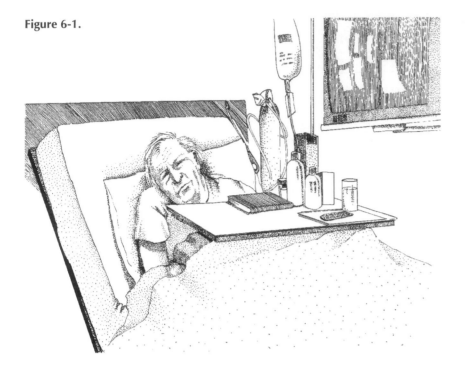

14. How will you address Frank's left neglect during his ADLs? What type of treatment activities would you use, and how would you set up his environment? Can you think of activities outside of the ADL routine to use as well?

15. How will you address Frank's dressing apraxia?

16. Please write out an instruction sheet for Frank to follow for his morning ADL routine.

17. Frank used to make his wife her morning coffee and breakfast of toast and cereal. Would this be a good treatment activity to do with Frank? Why or why not?

17a. You decide to do a kitchen activity with Frank. What safety measures would you want to follow?

18. Knowing Frank's hobbies and interests, would you be able to incorporate any of these into your treatment sessions? How would you go about this?

Equipment/Adaptations

19. Look at the illustration of Frank's hospital room (Figure 6-1). What changes would you make to Frank's room? Why?

Neuromusculoskeletal

20. What frame(s) of reference would you use to treat Frank's neuromusculoskeletal deficits?

21. Identify and prioritize the deficits in this area.

22. What treatment activities would you use to reduce the tone in Frank's UE and trunk?

23. How would you incorporate purposeful activity into your treatment plan?

NOTES

24. Frank has regained AROM of 15° in all motions of his UE. How would the treatment plan be modified? How would this affect his ability to use his UE functionally during ADLs and other activities?

25. Would you fabricate a splint for Frank's UE? If so, why and what type? If not, explain reasoning behind your decision. What would the wearing schedule be?

Cognition/Perception

26. In what ways will Frank's cognitive and perceptual deficits impact his daily functioning?

27. What functional activities would you use to address Frank's cognitive and perceptual deficits?
    fig-ground / wkst / memory cards
28. What adjunctive methods would you use to address Frank's cognitive and perceptual deficits?

Psychosocial

29. Frank uses humor throughout his treatment sessions, especially when he is having a particularly difficult time with something. Why do you think he is always trying to be funny, and how would you deal with it?

30. What concerns might Frank have relating to his loss of function?

31. What are some ways to support Frank psychologically to help him deal with his decreased abilities?

Patient/Family Education

32. Would you include Frank's wife in any patient/family education? If so, in what areas?

33. Using the areas identified in the question above, how would you go about educating Frank and his wife?

34. How will you work with the team in educating Frank on safety issues?

Situations

35. You walk into Frank's room in the morning to work with him on ADLs and find him in bed with the bedrails up, but trying to climb over them. He already has one leg over the bedrail and is trying to get his left leg over now. What do you do and why?

36. During a treatment session in the OT kitchen, Frank is making a cup of instant coffee. He turns on the stove, gets the kettle, and takes it to the sink to fill. He starts the water, notices a sponge, and starts to clean up the area around the sink, the sink itself, and the outside of the cabinets around the sink. He has forgotten the stove and the kettle, and has left the water running for 10 minutes during his cleaning. What do you think is the cause of this behavior and how would you refocus Frank? Would you adjust future kitchen activities and how?

37. Frank is in the middle of dressing himself. He has been following a set of cards with the steps for dressing on them with good results. Today Frank is not attending to the cards. He starts to get up to leave the room, but only has his boxers on; how do you redirect Frank to his dressing task?

38. During functional mobility Frank has progressed to ambulating with the hemi walker and supervision. However, he bumps into objects on his left side (the doorframe, the bed, the dresser, etc.). How will you address this during your treatment sessions?

NOTES

Discharge Planning

39. Frank is being discharged home. He now requires supervision for dressing and bathing using his cue cards and equipment. He continues to be impulsive and has poor insight into his deficits, and the carryover of new learning requires frequent repetitions. He can use his left UE to stabilize objects, but gross- and fine-motor coordination are still poor. He continues to have left neglect and has difficulty compensating for it. What services would you recommend for Frank and why?

40. Write a referral on Frank for the home care agency that will be treating him next.

41. What discharge instructions would you give Frank's wife?

NOTES

Chapter 7

Gloria:
Superficial, Partial-, and Full-Thickness Burns, 39% Total Body Surface Area

Gloria is a 44-year-old bilingual Hispanic woman with a diagnosis of burns to 39% of her body. She has superficial burns on 5% of her body, partial-thickness burns on 24% of her body, and full-thickness burns on 10% of her body. Gloria had suffered burns to both her hands, arms, anterior trunk, and neck area. The full-thickness burns are on the dorsum of her hands and posterior forearms. She also has a small area of partial-thickness burns on the forearms. Her trunk has partial-thickness burns, and the left side of her face has only superficial burns.

Gloria is a divorced mother of three. She owns her own 3-bedroom ranch-style house in a small suburb. She works as a chef for a large corporate catering firm. While at work, Gloria had set up the stovetop to begin preparing a meal. As she turned on the gas, the stovetop exploded into flames, burning Gloria severely. Luckily, she turned her face away quickly enough to avoid severe facial burns or inhalation injury. By looking at the location of Gloria's burns, you can see that she turned her head to the right and pulled her arms into the fetal position to protect her face.

Gloria was taken immediately to a hospital and transferred to the burn intensive care unit (ICU). She had been in the ICU and acute-care portion of the hospital for 4 weeks and was being transferred to the rehabilitation hospital for continued intensive therapy. She has skin grafts over her full-thickness burns. The grafts are autografts, taken from her left thigh. Because Gloria was in good health before her accident and a non-smoker, the doctors feel her partial-thickness burns are likely to heal themselves and have decided against grafting those areas. The doctors feel she is progressing well and is an excellent candidate for continued rehabilitation.

Gloria's three children (ages 14, 12, and 9) are staying with her sister while she is in the hospital. The two younger children visit Gloria often, while the older one is not able to stand being in the hospital and comes only occasionally. Gloria's employers have set up a worker's compensation case manager to oversee the treatment and hospital progress. Gloria's brother-in-law wants Gloria to sue. Gloria wants to get better and does not feel she can deal with the additional stress of a legal battle right now. Nonetheless, Gloria's sister, Tina, and her family have been supportive. Her ex-husband lives out-of-state and is remarried with his own family. Gloria's sister had called him to tell him about the accident. He offered no help other than to wish her a quick recovery. Gloria's parents are both living, but in poor health. They offer to do whatever they can to help out. Gloria's pastor is visiting her weekly for prayer. The plan is for Gloria to remain at the rehabilitation hospital until she is able to care for herself at home.

Occupational Therapy Evaluation

Gloria is seen for an occupational therapy evaluation the day after her rehab hospital admission. "Where have you been?" she asks. "The occupational therapist at the other hospital was in to see me right away. I need to get going to get home. Please help me." Gloria's eyes are sad and her voice is soft.

Gloria presents without any cognitive, visual, hearing, or perceptual deficits. She has sensory deficits on the dorsum and webbing of both hands, left side of face, posterior forearms, and anterior trunk related to the burns damaging the dermis. She also has sensory deficits in the left upper-arm area. Her skin in the damaged area is painful in some spots and not in others. The pigment is red and the skin is very taut and dry. The skin on her forearms is wrapped in bandages. The chart reveals that there are several "weepy" areas that are not healing well, making Gloria susceptible to infection.

Gloria has AROM WFL in her trunk and shoulders. Gloria's AROM is as follows for the left UE: elbow flexion: 110°; extension: −10°; wrist extension: 20°; wrist flexion: 25°; ulnar and radial deviation: 10°; supination: 45°; pronation: 60°; digits 2–5: MCP flexion: 80°; PIP/DIP flexion: 45°; digit extension: −10°; MCPs: −10° PIP/DIP; digit 1: opposition to lateral side of 3rd digit; MP flexion: 20°; IP flexion: 10°; thumb extension: −5°; palmar abduction: 15°; trace radial abduction. Gloria's AROM for the right UE is as follows: elbow flexion: 120°; extension: −5°; wrist extension: 25°; wrist flexion: 60°; ulnar and radial deviation: 10°; supination: 80° with pain; pronation: 85° with pain; digits 2–5: MCP flexion: 85°; PIP/DIP flexion: 55°; digit extension: −5°; MCP/PIP/DIPs digit 1: opposition to 4th digit; MP flexion: 25°; IP flexion: 15°; full thumb extension; palmar abduction: 25°; radial abduction: 15°. Gloria scored below the norm for the Jebsen Hand Function test.

Gloria is right-hand dominant. Her strength and coordination were not formally assessed but are obviously impaired due to the severity of her injuries. Gloria says she is in pain frequently and gets relief only from the medications.

Gloria is able to transfer to and from the bed and chair with minimal assistance. She has fallen once in the hospital after attempting to get up too quickly. Gloria needs assistance occasionally to turn in bed because of the pain. She ambulates without a device with contact guard. Gloria complains of pain in the left leg around the grafted area.

Gloria requires total assistance to bathe because of her fragile skin and the need for nursing to check her skin thoroughly and apply medication. Gloria is able to put on her own shoes (loafers), loose socks, and sweatpants. She has not been wearing a bra. She is able to put on a pullover shirt with minimal assistance. Gloria can do all of her oral hygiene herself, but usually asks for help because it "never feels clean enough" to her.

Gloria had been responsible for all the household duties and care of her children. She is still unable to perform those duties at this time. Gloria admits to feeling very upset about what happened. "God has mysterious plans for us. I just never thought he'd have this in mind for me," she remarks with sorrow.

Gloria agrees to participate in whatever treatment is necessary to get her home. She is to been seen by the physician, nursing, OT, PT, the dietitian, and social worker. She says her goals for herself are to take a shower and be able to take care of her daughters.

QUESTIONS

Goals/Treatment Plan

1. Devise a problem list for Gloria.

2. What are Gloria's strengths?

3. What short-term goals would you help Gloria to set for herself in regards to occupational therapy treatment?

4. What long-term goals would you and Gloria set for her occupational therapy treatment?

5. How might Gloria utilize those strengths to achieve her goals?

Safety/Precautions

6. What are the physical complications that may develop following severe burns? Explain in detail.

7. What are the precautions that should be taken to promote burn healing?

8. What are the signs of hypertrophic scarring?

9. What occupational therapy techniques can be used to prevent scar formation?

NOTES

Self-Care/Work/Leisure

10. Explain how you would organize an ADL session with Gloria, with the focus on teaching bathing techniques.

11. What precautions would you need to take to ensure Gloria's safety during an ADL retraining session?

12. Gloria tells you she feels like her clothes are "itching" her, and it is irritating for her to have anything touch her skin. Why might this be? How do you explain it to Gloria?

13. What can Gloria do to get relief from the situation in Question 12?

Equipment/Adaptations

14. What type of adaptive equipment might Gloria need to begin regaining independence in daily tasks?

15. What are the pros and cons of issuing adaptive equipment to a person in burn rehabilitation?

Neuromusculoskeletal

16. Write out a protocol of treatment focusing on desensitization treatment.

17. Write out a plan to restore Gloria's AROM.

18. Write out a plan for Gloria, focusing on hand strength and coordination.

19. How would you assess her strength and coordination on an ongoing basis?

Psychosocial

20. Gloria says she does not feel emotionally ready to even be in the OT room near the kitchen area. How do you respond to her request? Who might you tell about this?

21. What type of emotional impact do you think this injury has had on Gloria? On her family?

22. List the feelings Gloria has probably felt since her accident.

23. What professional discipline(s) could you recommend to help her deal with these issues?

24. Gloria has been praying with her pastor. How might a person's spirituality aid in the rehabilitation process?

Patient/Family Education

25. Gloria asks you to explain the scarring process to her. Write out what you would tell her.

Situations

26. The case manager from a worker's compensation agency asks you for documentation regarding Gloria's progress. What are you allowed to disclose, and what is confidential?

27. You are performing PROM with Gloria, and she is in obvious pain. She tells you to keep going. Do you? Why or why not?

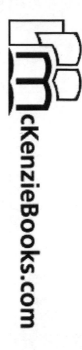

McKenzieBooks.com

Our return policy: Items are returnable within 14 days of the date you received the item. Any item returned must be in the exact same condition as when you received it. Please include this original packing slip with your return, and also please write the reason for returning the item on this packing slip. We will issue you a refund within 5 business days of receiving your returned item. Our return address is:

McKenzie Books, Returns Department
15370 SW Millikan Way
Beaverton, OR 97006-5138

Selling Back Your Books?
Visit us online at **Cash4Books.net** & find out how to get paid for your books FAST!

1-800-586-9581   -   orders@mckenziebooks.com   -   amazon.com/shops/mckenziebooks

Shipping Method: **USPS MediaMail**

Purchase Date: Mon, November 15, 2010

Order ID: **103-9332899-3866604**

Ship to: **Heather Hofmann**
1263 SW 15th Ave
ONTARIO, OREGON   97914-4227

Buyer Name: Heather Hofmann

SKU/ISBN	Qty	Title
GE03-4681 ISBN-13: 978-0781778398	**1**	**Mental Health Concepts and Techniques for the Occupational Therapy Assistant...**

NOTES

28. You are teaching Gloria how to care for her night hand splints. She tells you they hurt and the night nurse takes them off for her. This was the first you had heard of this. What do you do?

29. The weekend OT scheduled to see Gloria reports she refused Sunday treatment. When you ask Gloria, she says it is a day of rest and reflection. She asks not to be scheduled by OT or PT on Sundays. What do you think is more important, therapy or religion, and why?

30. Gloria's burns are healing well and she is now able to perform her bathing with only minimal assistance. She wants to go home for the holiday weekend and stay at her sister's overnight. Tina has agreed to assist her with ADLs. What education should you give Tina before Gloria goes on the leave of absence?

31. Before Gloria is ready to begin shower training, what things must you first teach her?

32. Gloria is still not feeling ready to begin any meal preparation tasks. Her daughters have offered to do the hot meal preparation at home. Should you continue to try to work toward independence in meal preparation using only the microwave? Why or why not?

Discharge Planning

33. Gloria's discharge plans are to return home and attend outpatient OT. What do you feel will be the goal of outpatient therapy?

34. Upon discharge, Gloria and her doctor ask you if you think she can now drive. What factors must be considered? What do you say?

35. Write up a home OT program for Gloria.

NOTES

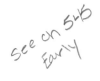

Chapter 8

Harris:
Spinal Cord Injury at T3, Complete

Harris is a 20-year-old African-American male with a diagnosis of complete spinal cord injury at T3 and resultant paraplegia. Harris also has a diagnosis of a fractured right tibia and fibula and right proximal radial and ulna fractures. Harris was admitted to the rehabilitation hospital from the acute-care hospital where he stayed for 2½ weeks after his accident.

Harris was in an automobile accident that resulted in his injuries. He was a passenger in the car and was struck from the right side by another car. Harris was pinned in the car for a short period of time and reports having no feeling in his legs immediately after the two cars collided. His friend, who was driving the car, was not seriously injured.

Harris lives with his fiancée, Marsha, on the 15th floor of a new apartment complex in the city. It is a small one-bedroom apartment. They intend to be married next spring. Harris is also planning on completing his baccalaureate degree in computer science and has one semester left to finish. Harris works full-time for his brother's plumbing business as a bookkeeper. During the little free time he has, he likes to travel with Marsha and golf with his friends. Harris had no functional deficits before the accident.

Harris' family is extremely supportive and visits daily. His brother Jeff calls frequently and his mother makes all his favorite meals, which she brings in for the nurses as well as Harris. Harris' father is not well and cannot visit as often due to respiratory distress, but telephones his son regularly. Marsha, who is a dental hygienist, has taken time off work to be with Harris every day at the hospital.

Harris is admitted to the rehabilitation hospital with the goal of returning home. He is eager to get started and tells the admission nurse "the more therapy, the better." Harris will be evaluated by PT, OT, nursing, social work, and the physiatrist.

Occupational Therapy Evaluation

Upon evaluation, Harris is talkative and motivated. He is in a wheelchair with lateral supports. His right UE is in a full-arm cast and his right LE is in a cast from the toes distal to the knee. Harris says he is right-handed. When asked how he has been feeling since the accident, his reply is "fine." When the question is rephrased as to his emotional state, his response is the same.

Harris has no cognitive, perceptual, visual, or hearing deficits. He has no sensation in either LE and reports no sensation in his buttocks as well. His UE sensation is intact, as is the sensation in his superior trunk region. His sensation is impaired in his inferior trunk region. Harris' low back area cannot be assessed during the evaluation due to his position in the chair.

Harris has no AROM in the LEs. His motion is intact in the left UE and cervical area. His right UE cannot be fully assessed due to the cast. Motion in his right digits is normal given the limitations of the cast. His left UE has normal strength; right UE is not fully assessed, but Harris can lift the cast up over his head.

Harris has no complaints of pain except for stiffness in his neck. He has some slight edema in the right digits at the MCP to DIP joints but no cyanosis. He has multiple bruises and abrasions over his body that nursing is monitoring.

Harris' sitting balance is poor to fair, and he is unable to sit up independently without minimal assistance. He does attempt to correct himself when leaning, but lacks the strength to maintain upright posture without external assistance. He is independent in sitting with the lateral supports in the wheelchair.

Harris uses a sliding board with moderate assistance to transfer from surface to surface. He is non-ambulatory and is non-weight-bearing on the right leg. Harris requires occasional assistance to propel himself in a wheelchair because of his inability to use his right arm. He performs bathing tasks ably and can wash his face, hands, chest, and peri-area independently. He requires total assistance for back, buttocks, and legs. He requires maximum assistance for dressing himself. Harris reports feeding himself without help although "it's messy sometimes." Harris has a catheter for urination and had been incontinent of bowel since the accident. His admission Functional Independence Measure (FIM) scores were in the 3 to 4 range for UE tables and 11 range for LE tables.

Harris wants to get started with therapy right away. He says his goals for rehabilitation are to "walk out of here and get on with my life."

QUESTIONS

Goals/Treatment Plan

1. What are your first thoughts when you hear Harris' goals?

2. What do you say in response?

3. What are Harris' problem areas?

4. What are Harris' strengths?

5. How could you incorporate his strengths into the treatment plan to help him meet his goals?

6. What short-term goals would you and Harris set for occupational therapy treatment?

7. What long-term goals would you and Harris set for occupational therapy treatment?

Safety/Precautions

8. What are some of your safety concerns for Harris given his condition?

9. How would the hospital staff go about addressing these issues?

10. What are the precautions that must be taken to provide Harris with proper preventative treatment measures?

Self-Care/Work/Leisure

11. Explain how you would set up an ADL session with Harris.

12. What precautions would you need to take to ensure his safety and success during ADL retraining?

13. Harris desperately wants to use a toilet on his own. What kinds of adaptations might make that more feasible for him?

14. What type of goals would you set for Harris' ADL skills once the casts are removed?

15. Harris' brother has told him not to worry about his job, but Harris keeps talking about it. Do you incorporate it into the treatment plan? If so, how?

16. Harris has refused to participate in any leisure activities at the hospital. "I'm here for work, not games," he says. What are your thoughts about this statement?

NOTES

Equipment/Adaptations

17. What type of adaptive equipment might improve Harris' independence while at the hospital?

18. What type of adaptive equipment might Harris need to function optimally at home?

Neuromusculoskeletal

19. What groups might be beneficial for Harris during his rehab stay?

20. Describe a treatment session focused on Harris' balance deficits.

21. Describe a treatment session focused on Harris' UE status while the cast is on his right arm.

22. Describe your UE treatment focus once the cast is removed at 8 weeks post-injury.

23. You see Harris in his room trying to do sit-ups in his bed. He is unable to do them, which only seems to make him try harder. What do you do in response to seeing this?

24. Physical therapy would like to co-treat with you for Harris' afternoon session. Describe what might be accomplished by having a co-treatment session with PT.

25. Describe what types of treatment might occur in a session co-treating with physical therapy.

26. Even though it is not in the occupational therapy realm of treatment, why is Harris' LE status important to occupational therapy?

Psychosocial

27. How does Harris appear to be coping with the accident and his injury?

28. What might be the impact of his accident on his relationship with his family?

29. What new issues will Harris' injury bring to his future with Marsha?

30. Even though Harris is not expressing such concerns, should they be addressed? If so, by whom?

Patient/Family Education

31. What type of education should Harris and his family receive regarding spinal cord injuries at the thoracic level?

32. What skills will Harris need to learn to incorporate into his daily routine in order to prevent self-injury? Find three agencies in your area that provide services for spinal cord individuals.

Situations

33. You are working with Harris in a co-treatment session with physical therapy. Harris still has no AROM in his LEs but has improved in his sitting balance and trunk strength. Harris asks the PT when she thinks he'll walk. The PT acts like she doesn't hear him, and he turns to you with the question. What do you say?

34. Explain how your response to the question above will impact Harris.

NOTES

35. Harris' friends from work come to visit him as he is ending an occupational therapy session. They start lifting the weights in the gym and showing off to one another. How might this make Harris feel? What do you say?

36. During an ADL session with Harris, you notice a small sore in the gluteal fold. What can be done to treat this problem? Why might it have occurred in the first place?

37. The doctor has cleared Harris to weight bear on his LEs. The PT wants to try the tilt table and asks you to help. Harris is excited and calls Marsha at home to come see him. Marsha arrives at the hospital while Harris is strapped in the table in an upright position. She tries to be positive but starts to cry. Harris demands to be put back in the chair and is obviously shaken by her reaction. What do you do and say to Marsha? To Harris? To the treatment team?

38. How might the events in the question above affect Harris in the future?

39. Harris continues to show improvement through his determination. He is performing the sliding board transfers and ADLs in bed independently. He wants to be able to shower alone. How can you help him achieve this goal? Explain.

40. Harris wants to be continent of bowel and bladder before he leaves the hospital. The catheter has been removed but he still is not continent all the time due to motor and sensory loss. What can you do to help Harris achieve his goals of continence?

Discharge Planning

41. Harris plans to go home soon. What questions should you ask him to assist with the transition back to the community?

42. What equipment would you order for Harris to be sent to his apartment?

43. What type of teaching would need to be done with Marsha before Harris goes home?

44. What type of wheelchair would you and the PT order for Harris to take home? Be specific and include cost and payor source.

45. Harris wants to return to work. How long do you think it will be before he is able to do that?

46. What will need to be in place before Harris returns to work?

47. Harris has also spoken of returning to school since he has only one semester left. What will he need to investigate prior to his return to the college?

48. What resources might there be at the college to support Harris' return to his academics?

49. Harris is going to continue with rehabilitation through the Visiting Nurse Association until he can arrange outpatient treatment. What would you recommend the home OT to work on?

NOTES

Chapter 9

Ingrid:
Traumatic Brain Injury— Ranchos Level V

Ingrid is a 45-year-old Caucasian woman who suffered a traumatic brain injury from a skiing accident. She had been on a skiing vacation in the northwest with her husband and two children: a son, age 15, and a daughter, age 8. She lost control and tumbled several hundred feet down the mountain before hitting a tree and coming to a stop. During the tumble, her head hit the ground several times. She was not wearing a helmet. The ski patrol got to the scene within 10 minutes and found Ingrid unconscious. She was transported to the local hospital where she was stabilized and then taken by helicopter to a large hospital that could deal with her head trauma. She spent several weeks in the acute-care hospital, which was near the ski resort, several hundred miles from her home. She was discharged to a rehabilitation hospital near her home in the city for further therapy and so that her family could visit and be an active part of her rehabilitation.

Prior to the accident, Ingrid was a social worker in a skilled nursing facility. She had no deficits in any occupational performance area. She was active in her daughter's school, volunteering to help out with reading in the classroom and on other school committees. She and her family live in a two-story colonial home in a suburban neighborhood. Her husband, Tom, works as an accountant for a small accounting firm. He took a lot of time off immediately after the accident to stay near Ingrid's hospital, which was far from the family's home. Their two children returned home and Tom's parents stayed with them. Tom is afraid to take more time off from work. The family needs the income and health benefits, and the tax season is approaching. Their financial situation will be tight without Ingrid's income. She has no disability insurance.

The plan is that Ingrid will be discharged to her home in 6 weeks. She is being seen by occupational therapy, physical therapy, speech therapy, social work, nursing, and various physician specialties.

Occupational Therapy Evaluation

OT evaluation reveals Ingrid to be at Ranchos Level V—confused inappropriate. She responds to simple directions, but is highly distractible, has poor short-term memory, and has little carryover for new learning from one session to the next. She has intact sensation, vision, and hearing. Perceptual processing is impaired for spatial relations, categorization, and position in space.

Her physical status presents with mild to moderate increased tone (proximal to distal) in her UEs, with the left side worse than the right. She has PROM in her left shoulder of 0–85° flexion, 0–50° external rotation, 0–80° internal rotation. Her UE PROM in the right shoulder is 0–105° flexion, 0–70° external rotation, 0–80° internal rotation, 0–40° horizontal abduction, 0–90° horizontal adduction. PROM in remainder is WFL. AROM is less than 1/2 normal AROM in both shoulders. She also has mild increased tone in her trunk and moderate tone in her LEs. She continues to demonstrate some primitive reflexes, especially ATNR, and she has decreased equilibrium and righting reactions. Her coordination is impaired due to the tone in her UEs. Ingrid is right-handed.

Ingrid requires minimum physical assistance and frequent verbal cues for all transfers and wheelchair mobility. She is currently non-ambulatory. She requires moderate assistance with all ADL tasks due to her physical and cognitive deficits. Ingrid currently has little insight into her deficits. She talks about her family and her children and misses them a lot. She brightens up when they visit and returns to her room and lies on her bed once they leave. She has expressed anger at the staff and feels she is being kept a prisoner against her wishes. She lacks initiation and when in group situations says whatever is on her mind, even if it is a criticism of another patient or staff member. She has alienated a few staff and patients by calling them "fat," "stupid," or "ugly," among other things.

When asked what her goals are, Ingrid only states "to get out of this place and back to my own home." Tom is hopeful that Ingrid can improve enough to return home, drive, and take care of the kids.

QUESTIONS

Goals/Treatment Plan

1. Write a list of problems that need to be addressed by OT during Ingrid's 6-week expected rehab stay. Prioritize them based on her and Tom's goals.

2. What are Ingrid's strengths?

3. Based on the problem list from Question 1, write long- and short-term goals.

4. Given Ingrid's level of cognitive function, how will you make your goals client-centered?

5. How will you include Ingrid's family in your treatment plan?

6. What role will other team members have in meeting Ingrid's rehab needs? What role would a COTA have in treatment planning and implementation?

Safety/Precautions

7. What safety issues do you need to be aware of with Ingrid?

8. How will you collaborate with other staff in addressing Ingrid's safety issues?

Self-Care/Work/Leisure

9. Given Ingrid's motor, cognitive, perceptual, and interpersonal deficits, what methods would you use to address her self-care deficits?

10. Ingrid is able to brush her teeth and wash her hands and face at the sink from the wheelchair with set-up. What would you address next in the bathing/grooming performance area? How would you go about this?

11. Would you teach Ingrid to use adaptive equipment for her ADL routine? Please explain your answer.

12. You want to do a kitchen activity with Ingrid. What activity would you choose and how would you organize it to ensure her success?

13. What types of simple home-management tasks would you work on with Ingrid?

14. What types of leisure activities would you try with Ingrid, and why did you choose these?

Equipment/Adaptations

15. Tom is looking toward the day when Ingrid returns home. What environmental modifications, either temporary or permanent, would you suggest he make knowing the type of home they live in?

16. What type of modifications might you need to make to Ingrid's wheelchair, and what pieces of adaptive equipment would you give to her so that she can carry her memory aids?

NOTES

Neuromusculoskeletal

17. Ingrid's coordination is impaired for gross- and fine-motor activities. Please address her sitting position and describe why correct sitting position is an important component for coordination.

18. After you position Ingrid correctly, what techniques will you use to normalize her muscle tone, and what areas of her UE will you start with?

19. Please describe some functional treatment activities that you would use to help normalize muscle tone.

20. Physical therapy and occupational therapy work closely in the area of normalizing muscle tone. How will you ensure that your treatment is different from physical therapy's treatment?

Cognition/Perception

21. Given Ingrid's Ranchos level, what types of purposeful treatment activities would you do to work on her cognitive deficits?

22. What type of structure, if any, would Ingrid benefit from to compensate for her cognitive deficits? Given Ingrid's perceptual problems, what key areas could you expect to be impacted the most and why?

Psychosocial

23. Ingrid gets easily frustrated during her treatment sessions. How would you deal with this issue? Ingrid frequently gets angry at her family during their visits. How would you assist her family to understand these outbursts? Are there strategies they could use to minimize these outbursts?

23a. What affect do you think Ingrids accident will have on her role as mother and spouse? How might OT address these changes?

Patient/Family Education

24. Ingrid has progressed to a Level VI on the Ranchos Scale in her cognitive function. She requires a wheelchair for mobility when she is fatigued, and uses a large base quad cane with supervision at other times. She is going to be discharged home. What safety issues would you want to educate her family about?

24a. What support services exist in your community for patients and families with TBI? Which one might Ingrid benefit from and why?

Situations

25. Ingrid is taking a shower for the first time with OT. She is very distractible, has a short attention span, and little insight. How would you structure the task so that it is successful and not frustrating for Ingrid?

26. Ingrid has always worn tailored clothing in the latest style. This may involve a skirt, blouse and jacket, fitted slacks, nylons, and attractive shoes. She wears jeans and casual sweaters for relaxation, with comfortable shoes. Tom wants to know if he should bring these types of clothes from home, or if he should go out and buy coordinated sweatsuits and sneakers. What do you tell him, and what is the reasoning for your answer?

27. Ingrid is in a grooming group with three other women. She attends well for the first 5 minutes and then starts asking if she can leave. If she isn't allowed to leave, she begins to talk to the other women and distracts them. The group is a part of her treatment plan, and she is supposed to attend. How would you deal with Ingrid's behavior?

NOTES

28. Every time Ingrid's children come to visit her she starts crying and asks them to take her out of this prison. They have come during one of your OT sessions, and she is distracted by their presence. You are working with Ingrid on some simple cognitive activities (games, pegboards, etc.). Is there a way that you could incorporate their presence into your treatment session?

29. Ingrid goes home for a day with her husband. When she returns, he reports that she was not able to remember where anything was in the house, even which room was her bedroom. He is quite upset about this and is not sure how realistic he has been about her recovery. What do you tell him?

Discharge Planning

30. What services would you recommend for Ingrid on her discharge from the rehab hospital if she were at a Ranchos Level VI or VII? How would they differ and why?

31. What services would you recommend for Ingrid? Do you think she would benefit better from therapy in outpatient or home care? Why?

32. Write a discharge referral for Ingrid.

NOTES

Chapter 10

Jing:
Right Above Elbow Amputation

Jing is a 27-year-old Chinese man who suffered a long right above-elbow (AE) amputation following an industrial accident in the workplace. He is a paper cutter at a printing plant, managing a large industrial paper cutter that cuts huge stacks of paper to size following printing. He was preparing a stack of papers to be cut when the machine malfunctioned and came down before Jing could get his arm out of the way. He was rushed to the hospital where immediate measures were taken to stop the bleeding and close the stump. He was not a candidate for limb reattachment.

Jing has been working at his job for 3 years since arriving in this country. He emigrated here and was given asylum for being a Chinese dissident. He lives in a large city. He has been going to school in the evenings to learn English and hopes to enter college in another year, when his English has improved. Jing has no family in the area. He does not drive, relying on public transportation and a bicycle to get around. He has developed a few close Chinese friends from his English-as-a-second-language classes, and they go out after class and hang out on the weekends.

Jing lives in a one-bedroom apartment in the city with two other Chinese men, as they cannot afford a bigger place. They take turns cooking and shopping at the neighborhood Chinese market. They continue to eat traditional Chinese food and maintain traditional Chinese values and customs.

Jing is a quiet man of few words but with deep feelings about his country. He becomes quite animated when engaged in conversation about China and his "work" there. He was a student in China working on a degree in engineering when he left to seek asylum. He does not express his emotions often, but values his intelligence and his goal of achieving an education in this country. Jing would love to return to China someday. He worries about the family he left behind and how they are being treated since his fleeing.

Jing was admitted to a rehabilitation hospital in a nearby city because they specialize in amputations and trauma. He is 2 weeks post-amputation at the time of his rehabilitation hospital admission. He is to be seen by occupational therapy, physical therapy, nursing, social work, and dietary.

Occupational Therapy Evaluation

Jing's English comprehension is fair, but he doesn't understand medical terms. He speaks broken English and has a difficult time expressing himself. His English reading comprehension is poor. Jing demonstrates no deficits in cognition, perception, hearing, or vision. He does present with hypersensitivity of the stump. He is a right-handed man with AROM of the left UE WNL, and the right shoulder WNL as well. His muscle strength in both shoulders is very good, as he is in good physical shape from lifting heavy paper bundles. He has edema in the stump, which is wrapped daily. His surgical wound is still healing, but the stitches have been removed. He experiences both phantom pain and phantom limb phenomenon in his right UE and is having a difficult time dealing with this.

Jing is independent in bed mobility using a trapeze or the bed rails. He transfers with stand-by assistance for safety. He requires minimum to moderate assistance for bathing and dressing. Both dynamic and static balance are good for sitting and standing. He is feeding himself, using his left hand with setup, and his food is cut for him. He feels very clumsy and gets frustrated at meals.

Jing is having a difficult time adjusting to the fact that he has lost his arm, as shown by his gestures and facial expressions. However, he does not like to talk about his feelings. He participates in occupational therapy, but is despondent and does not take an active role.

Jing was fitted for his preparatory mechanical prosthesis and training is about to start with it; he does not show much enthusiasm about it at the moment. He has expressed the feelings that without his arm he is not a whole person and therefore not useful to society, and fears a woman will not want him without his being "whole."

It has been difficult to elicit goals from Jing, partly due to a language barrier and partly due to his despondency. He just says to "do what you think is best."

Questions

Goals/Treatment Plan

1. Given Jing's despondency, how will you include him in your goal-setting and treatment-planning process?

2. Write a problem list for Jing.

3. What is the purpose of the preparatory mechanical prosthesis, and what are your goals in relation to the prosthesis?

4. Given that this was a work-related injury, what insurance do you think would cover Jing's rehabilitation? How will this affect his length of stay and your treatment plan?

5. What impact does Jing's cultural background have on your treatment plan and your method of working with him?

6. Write a treatment plan for Jing.

7. What part of the treatment plan is it appropriate for a COTA to be doing?

8. Using the Model of Human Occupation, what do you see as Jing's strengths and deficits in the volitional and habituation subsystems?

Safety/Precautions

9. What safety issues should you be aware of with Jing?

10. What precautions should you remember regarding Jing's stump and wound?

Self-Care/Work/Leisure

11. What functional activities will you start with when teaching Jing to use his prosthesis for ADLs? Why did you choose these activities?

12. Jing is very frustrated at meals because he is so clumsy with his left hand, and he isn't proficient at using his prosthesis at mealtimes. What types of suggestions would you have to assist him in this area?

13. What skills does Jing need in order to return to school?

14. How would you incorporate fine-motor coordination training into a leisure activity?

15. You want to work on meal preparation with Jing. What type of meal would you think appropriate?

NOTES

Equipment/Adaptations

16. What equipment would you recommend for Jing to assist him with returning to school?

17. Since Jing relied heavily on bicycle transportation to get around, what training and adaptations will he need for his bicycle?

Neuromusculoskeletal

18. How would you train Jing to flex and extend the elbow joint of his prosthesis?

19. What type of exercises would you give Jing to do before he begins training with his prosthesis?

20. Jing complains of phantom pain and phantom limb sensations. What type of treatment would you use to address these issues?

21. How would you begin training Jing in the use of the terminal device of his prosthesis? What type of terminal device would be most appropriate for him? What type of functional activities would you use in training him to use the terminal device?

Psychosocial

22. What psychological supports can you identify for Jing at the rehabilitation hospital?

23. What value does the Chinese culture place on individuals with handicaps or amputations? How might this affect Jing's attitude toward his disability?

24. Given Jing's initial despondency and feelings of "not being whole," how will you approach your treatment sessions with him?

25. What supports do you think he might need upon his discharge and how would you set them up?

25a. Jing is worried about how he will support himself when he is discharged. In what ways can OT address this area?

Patient/Family Education

26. Find a website that you feel would be a good source of information and support for Jing. Why do you feel this is a good site for Jing?

27. What patient education issues can you identify for Jing, and how would you address them?

Situations

28. You enter Jing's room one day to begin a treatment session, and you find him sitting on his bed with his prosthesis in his lap, crying. He tells you that he doesn't feel life is worth living if he has to use a prosthesis for the rest of his life. How do you respond to him, and what do you do?

29. Jing's primary language is Chinese. He speaks and comprehends English to a degree, but the stress of his condition and the new medical terms have made communication with him difficult. He will nod his head as if he understands your instructions, but then is not able to do what you have instructed. How can you overcome this language barrier during therapy?

NOTES

Discharge Planning

30. Jing is scheduled to return to his old apartment with his old roommates in 1 week. He has become proficient enough to use his prosthesis for ADLs and IADLs, but he is concerned about how his roommates will make the environmental adjustments that need to be made to the apartment. What activities can you do with him during your last week that will help him to prepare for this?

31. Jing is being discharged home. His current status is dressing with sweat pants and pull over tops. He has elastic laces on his shoes and struggles to get socks on. He feeds himself using his right, but is slow and he does not trust using a computer yet. His strength in his right shoulder is good, and he is able to wear the prosthesis for 5 hours a day. Write a discharge note for continual OT upon his return home.

NOTES

Part IV

Transitional Care Unit

Chapter 11

Kim:
Coronary Artery Bypass Graft x3,
Congestive Heart Failure

Kim is a 63-year-old African-American single female. She underwent a coronary artery bypass graft (CABG) x3 2 weeks ago. Kim had been experiencing chest pain with minimal exertion and was diagnosed with three blocked coronary arteries. She underwent the CABG procedure at a large teaching hospital. She has additional diagnoses of congestive heart failure, diabetes, hypothyroidism, and schizophrenia. Recovery has been unremarkable from a medical perspective.

Prior to her procedure, she was living in her second floor walk-up apartment in the suburbs with her parrot, Cleo, and her dog, Casey. Kim has never been married. There are no laundry facilities in the apartment building. Kim works part-time as a clerk in a convenience store, which includes moving boxes, stocking the shelves, and managing the cash register. She attends a day hospital program 2 days a week, as well. She takes medication for her schizophrenia and does well as long as she stays on her medication. She drives short distances for errands.

Kim has been independent in all her life tasks, although the few months prior to her surgery she started to tire easily and was not able to do as much as usual. She has an older sister who lives far away and is unable to travel to be with her. Kim has few friends. She does not go out much socially and has a very limited support system. She is a quiet person and has difficulty making friends, not feeling comfortable in social situations. Kim loves animals, and her pets are like her family. She dotes on both animals, buying them special treats, taking Casey on walks with Cleo on her shoulder. She worries about her animals while she is on the transitional care unit. She is planning on returning home to her pets and hopes to return to work and to the day program. She is being seen by occupational therapy, physical therapy, and daily nursing care. Her length of stay is expected to be 2 weeks.

Occupational Therapy Evaluation

Kim wears bifocal glasses. Her hearing, sensation, and perception are all intact. She appears to be forgetful about recent information.

Her AROM in both UEs is WFL. Her strength is 3 + /5 throughout both UE. She has no deficits in coordination and is right-handed. Her endurance is poor for all functional activities. She continues to have pain (6 on a scale of 1 to 10) in the sternum. She fatigues easily, however, and only tolerates 30 minutes out of bed at a time. She has pain from the incision on her chest. Her skin is intact, except for the surgical site, which is healing well.

She can roll in bed using the siderails and can only move from sit to supine by first raising the head of the bed. She transfers from sit to stand with the moderate assist of one, and is ambulating using a rolling walker due to LE weakness. Kim has refused to dress in anything more than a hospital gown. She will wash her hands and face sitting up in bed, but then is too tired to continue and allows the staff to complete her bathing. Kim is eating very little and claims not to have much appetite.

She has expressed to all staff that her goals are to return home to her animals. She is willing to participate in treatment, but just "doesn't have the energy."

QUESTIONS

Goals/Treatment Plan

1. Using the Model of Human Occupation, how would you assess Kim's volitional and habituation subsystems?

2. Make a problem list for Kim, and put the problems in priority according to her goals.

3. Write the long- and short-term goals for the first three problems on your problem list.

4. What treatment methods and activities will you plan in order to achieve your short-term goals?

5. What part of the treatment planning process can a COTA participate in? What aspects of this treatment plan could a COTA carry out?

6. What are the psychosocial issues for Kim? How will you incorporate the psychosocial issues into your treatment plan?

6a. What type of treatment groups would Kim benefit from?

Safety/Precautions

7. Kim's blood pressure and pulse should be monitored during therapy for what reasons?

8. At what blood pressure reading would you stop activity? How long would you wait to see if her blood pressure came down? What would you do in regards to notifying other team members of a high blood pressure reading?

9. Other than pulse and blood pressure, what other precautions should you be aware of?

Self-Care/Work/Leisure

10. How would you address Kim's bathing skills? Describe how you would grade the activity and progress her from her current level to being able to bathe seated at the sink.

11. Since Kim is planning to return home, what type of kitchen activity would you plan for your first session in the kitchen? Why? What are the basal metabolic equivalents (MET) for this task?

12. Your facility is set up with a washer and dryer in the OT area. What type of energy-conservation techniques will you teach Kim to accomplish this task without getting tired?

13. What part of the dressing task do you think would be most difficult for Kim to accomplish and why? Do you think Kim's surgery will affect her ability to perform this job? If so, how?

Equipment/Adaptations

14. How will you recommend that Kim adapt her daily morning routine to account for her poor endurance?

15. What techniques should Kim be taught to help her manage her energy during her recovery?

16. Will you recommend any adaptive equipment for Kim to take home? If so, what and why?

17. How will you address Kim's bed mobility issues in therapy?

NOTES

Neuromusculoskeletal

18. Write out an exercise program using theraband to improve Kim's UE strength. How will you document this so it pertains to OT?

19. Describe two craft activities that you could do to increase Kim's endurance. How would you set these up? Why did you choose them? Did you consider Kim's interests in planning them?

Cognition/Perception

20. Kim is having difficulty remembering recent information. What compensatory techniques can you use to address this issue?

21. What types of adjunctive activities can you use to address her memory issue? How would you transfer this training to functional activities?

Psychosocial

22. Given what you know about Kim's psychological status, how well do you think she is coping with her current condition? What would you do to assist her in this area?

22a. What concerns do you have in relation to her Schizophrenia?

23. Kim has consistently expressed a desire to go home and to return to work, but is just as consistently not making progress in therapy. She continues to complain of fatigue and feeling too tired to participate. How would you deal with this issue, and what other team members might you confer with?

Patient/Family Education

24. Your supervisor has asked you to help develop an educational group for patients who have undergone the CABG procedure. Each discipline (OT, nursing, PT, social work, nutrition) will lead a 1-hour session. What would you do for the OT session and why?

25. What type of patient education material would you give to Kim and why?

26. Please find two websites that would be of benefit to Kim. Why did you choose these?

Situations

27. Kim has no clothing at the transitional care unit, and you would like to start working on dressing skills. She does not want to ask anyone to bring in clothes from her apartment, even though there is a neighbor who has a key to her apartment. How would you address this issue?

28. You are in the middle of working on showering with Kim one morning. She starts to complain of chest pain and shortness of breath. She stops washing, catches her breath, and resumes the activity. After a few minutes, she again gets short of breath, but doesn't complain of chest pain. What should you do?

29. Kim keeps forgetting to pace herself during her ADL routine. Every time you work with her, you must remind her that she has to slow down. If she continues at the pace she sets, she gets short of breath and has to rest. How do you handle this situation?

30. During an exercise group, you notice that Kim is making comments as though she is talking to someone else in the room. She seems distracted and unable to focus on the exercise. You ask her who she is talking to, and she tells you she is talking to her mother. What do you do?

NOTES

Discharge Planning

31. Kim has progressed enough that she is able to return home. She is now able to wash at the sink while seated, and can tolerate being out of bed for up to 4 hours. She has improved UE muscle strength to 4/5. She can make a light meal (toast, coffee, sandwich) using energy-conservation techniques. She can put on a hospital gown, but still hasn't addressed getting fully dressed because she had no clothing. Write up a referral for continued occupational therapy in home care.

32. Based on the above description of Kim's status at discharge, which of the initial long-term goals that you set have been achieved? What might have been reasons that your other goals were not met?

NOTES

Chapter 12

Lyle: Right Total Knee Replacement

Lyle is a 57-year-old African-American male with a diagnosis of a right total knee replacement. Lyle has a past medical history that includes morbid obesity, coronary artery disease, and hypertension. Lyle had elective knee replacement surgery due to pain in the right knee and decreased mobility.

Prior to the surgery, Lyle was independent with all self-care using several adaptive devices including a reacher, a long-handled shoehorn, and a hand-held shower hose. He was independent in home management and community mobility skills. He ambulated with a limp, but used no device. Lyle works full-time as an account representative for a corporation that manufactures institutional kitchen equipment. Lyle's job requires much travel, and he spends most of his time in the car and on the telephone. He reports that his job takes most of his time and that he works close to 60 hours per week, including all his travel time. With his company's recent downsizing, he now covers an even larger geographic area, but he "dares not complain" for fear of losing his job. He says he only has a few more years until retirement and plans to keep working until then. Lyle is very concerned about the amount of time he has to lose from work due to the surgery and hopes to get back as soon as he is able. He says, laughing nervously, "I don't want to give them a chance to realize they'd be better off without me."

Lyle is divorced with three grown children. His youngest daughter, Chloe, moved in with him recently following her own divorce. She also works full-time and attends college part-time in the evenings. Lyle lives in a two-story condominium where the bedrooms and bathroom are on the second floor. Lyle says he wants to move somewhere that has everything on one floor, but the condominium is so convenient to his office that he just can't bear to drive any more during the day than he has to.

Lyle is a very large man, standing 5' 10" tall and weighing close to 300 pounds. His lifestyle is hectic and he admits to doing little to take care of himself. He claims he has no time for exercising or eating right. His physician has been trying to get him to lose weight for a while, with little luck. Although he has always been overweight, Lyle has actually been putting on weight recently. He felt it is due to longer time spent in the car, his sedentary lifestyle, stress related to his work, and his recent divorce from his wife of 31 years. He says he realizes the excess weight is what has expedited the deterioration of the right knee. His plan is to return to his current living situation and to work as soon as he is capable of doing so.

Lyle had right knee replacement surgery on May 7th and was sent to the transitional care unit on May 9th. His surgery was uncomplicated, and it is anticipated that he will be at the unit for rehabilitation for 1 to 1½ weeks. His HMO case manager has planned for him to continue his therapy on an outpatient basis once he returns home. Lyle will have involvement from PT, OT, nursing, nutritionist, and social service.

Occupational Therapy Evaluation

Upon evaluation, Lyle is cooperative and talkative. He presents with no cognitive, perceptual, sensory, visual, or hearing deficits. He has functional use of both UEs; however, the ROM in his shoulders is limited slightly by his large body mass. He has no coordination or strength deficits and is right-hand dominant.

Lyle has a great deal of pain in the right knee. He gets relief from the pain medication and takes the maximum dosage allowed daily. He complains of a dull pain when he is not moving and of excruciating pain in the right knee during all right LE motion. His knee is edematous and red, and the incision is covered with a dressing that nursing changes twice a day. Lyle is being watched closely for any signs of infection or deep vein thrombosis.

The mobility portion of the OT evaluation is completed with the physical therapist in case two people are needed to assist. Lyle is able to roll independently in the bed with the use of the bed rails. He requires minimum assistance to sit up from supine. He wears a knee immobilizer on the right leg to stabilize it during transfers. He is allowed touch down weight-bearing on the right leg and is to wear the knee immobilizer at all times except during exercises and while using the continuous passive motion machine. Lyle transfers from bed to chair with moderate assistance and performs commode transfers with the maximum assist of one, needing help with managing his clothing. Lyle uses a standard walker for all transfers. At this time, he is not walking, only performing stand-pivot transfers from one place to another. He fatigues quickly after the transfers. Shower transfers are not attempted during the evaluation. Lyle uses a wheelchair and can propel it independently.

Lyle is able to feed and groom himself, as well as dress and bathe his upper body independently. He requires maximum assistance for all lower body care. He cannot reach his right foot while wearing the knee immobilizer and admits that this was hard for him to do even before the surgery. He is unable to perform any kitchen or home management tasks at the time of the evaluation.

Lyle is eager to begin therapy and agrees to participate in "whatever I need to do to go home." Lyle states his goals for occupational therapy are to shower and dress himself and be able to make coffee. His only stipulation to participation is that the therapist coordinate with the nurse to be sure he has his pain medication **before** he is expected to do any kind of therapy. "I'd like to have as little pain as possible!" he remarks.

QUESTIONS

Goals/Treatment Plan

1. Write out a problem list for Lyle.

2. Write out a list of Lyle's strengths.

3. What goals would you and Lyle set for his occupational therapy treatment?

4. What difficulties might you anticipate in Lyle meeting his goals?

5. How might you collaborate with other team members to incorporate OT goals into Lyle's program at the transitional care unit?

6. Write out a specific treatment plan for Lyle, including frequency.

Safety/Precautions

7. What are some safety issues that might arise for Lyle?

8. How could you work with Lyle and the other team members to reduce the safety risk?

9. What are the precautions for a total knee replacement?

Self-Care/Work/Leisure

10. How would you prepare Lyle to perform his ADLs given his knee replacement?

11. What portion of the ADL tasks do you anticipate will be most difficult for Lyle to accomplish?

12. How might you adapt this portion of the ADL routine to maximize independence?

13. How would you design a session with Lyle to prepare a light snack using the microwave?

NOTES

14. What part of the snack preparation would you anticipate to be the most difficult for Lyle? Why?

15. Lyle reports feeling bored on the unit since he's not used to "doing nothing." How would you address his leisure needs?

16. At what level will Lyle be able to return to work?

17. How long do you anticipate it will take him to accomplish this?

Equipment/Adaptations

18. What type of adaptive equipment would Lyle need to maximize his independence?

19. Given that his estimated length of stay is 1 to 1½ weeks, what equipment might Lyle need at home to maximize independence?

20. Explain how you would go about ordering such equipment for Lyle, keeping in mind he has an HMO for his insurer.

21. Given what you know about Lyle's living situation, what adaptations might need to be made at his home for him to function?

22. What questions could you ask to determine if Lyle might need adaptation equipment at work?

23. What adaptations to his lifestyle might Lyle have to make to return to work?

Neuromusculoskeletal

24. What would you do within the realm of OT to address Lyle's neuromusculoskeletal status?

Psychosocial

25. What coping strategies is Lyle using to deal with his recent surgery?

26. What concerns do you think Lyle has regarding his temporary functional limitations?

27. What are some ways to support Lyle psychologically to help him deal with his decreased mobility and function?

Patient/Family Education

28. What type of instruction does Lyle need to promote recovery?

29. How might you involve Lyle's family to help him meet his goals?

30. In what ways could OT assist Lyle in fitting exercise into his daily routine?

Situations

31. You enter Lyle's room and find him trying to get to the bathroom by himself without the knee immobilizer on. What might you say to him, and what would you do?

32. Lyle tells you he was trying to get to the bathroom alone because two nursing assistants already came in and told him to wait a minute, and he'd been waiting for almost 40 minutes. How would you respond to his comment?

NOTES

33. Would you address his statement with any other staff members? Why?

34. If you did decide to address it with someone, who would it be, and what might the response/ramifications be?

35. You enter Lyle's room at 8:30 A.M. to begin an ADL treatment. Lyle tells you he still has not had his 7:00 A.M. pain medication and cannot start until at least 30 minutes **after** he's had it. You have a busy morning with other ADL treatments and cannot reschedule him later. What do you do?

36. You again set a time to see Lyle and his pain medication is not given to him prior to therapy as it is supposed to be. Lyle refuses therapy again and is angry about the situation. What do you do?

37. You are with Lyle in the therapy gym, and he begins to complain of pain in the left LE. How might that be explained?

38. Who would you speak to about Lyle's left leg pain?

Discharge Planning

39. When would you begin discharge planning with Lyle?

40. What would you need to review with Lyle's daughter Chloe before he returns home?

41. What would you do if Lyle decided 2 days before the planned discharge date that he was leaving to go home? What factors may have led him to make that decision?

42. If you felt Lyle was not ready to leave, what course of action might you take? What would you say to Lyle?

43. What level of function would you feel Lyle would need to be at to be discharged home safely?

44. Would you recommend continued OT services for Lyle after discharge? Explain why or why not.

45. Write out a home program for Lyle.

NOTES

Chapter 13

Mary:
Left Total Hip Replacement,
Osteoarthritis

Mary is a 72-year-old Caucasian female of Italian descent with a diagnosis of a left hip replacement. Mary also has osteoarthritis, hypertension, and a history of urinary tract infections. Mary had elective replacement surgery at the urging of her orthopedic surgeon. Mary had been suffering with progressively worse pain in the left hip over the past 2 years and had finally decided she could not tolerate it any further. She had canceled the surgery once before, thinking she could do without it.

Mary has been becoming noticeably less active because of the hip pain for the last 8 months. Prior to hospitalization, Mary had been independent in all ADLs and home and community management. She did state, however, that it has been taking her much longer to do her morning routine and all daily tasks because of the hip pain. She had been able to ambulate without a device until approximately 2 months ago, when she decided to borrow a cane from her sister and use it "to lean on." She also found herself going upstairs only when she had to, such as to use the bathroom. Mary admits to cutting down on her coffee in the morning to help keep the trips to the bathroom to a minimum. Mary lives alone in the suburbs in her own home, which has five stairs to enter and 12 stairs to the second floor where the bedroom and bathroom are. She has never been married and has no children. Mary has a sister who lives within walking distance from her home, but Mary says she started driving over recently instead of walking the two blocks for the visit.

Mary had moved to the United States 55 years ago from Italy. She had been a nanny and a preschool teacher most of her career and had retired 7 years ago at the age of 65. She had been socially active prior to her surgery. She plays cribbage once a week with three other women and is a volunteer at the town library where she conducts children's reading and story hours. She is very distressed that the story times are going to be canceled because of her surgery and spoke with hostility of the others at the library for not filling in while she is in the hospital. Mary is a very kind woman with a strong sense of right and wrong. She speaks frequently about how wrong it is to allow the children to go without their stories and how wrong it is for the others at the library to be so selfish. Mary seems to have a hard time letting go of feelings that bother her, and she deals with it by talking about it with anyone who will listen. She can often be seen telling the housekeepers and dietary aides as they enter and exit her room about the inconsideration of the other library volunteers. Mary seems to use her issue of choice to avoid conversations regarding her surgery.

Mary had an uncomplicated total hip replacement surgery. The acetabulum and femoral head and neck were replaced using a posterolateral approach. Mary has had no complications from her surgery and was moved from the acute portion of the hospital to the transitional care unit after 3 days. Mary had initially hoped she would be able to go home directly after surgery. She agreed to move onto the transitional care unit after she and her sister realized that she would not be able to be at home safely. Her discharge plans are to return home with services in 1 to 2 weeks. Mary will be followed at the transitional care unit by the physiatrist in charge. Her team will include PT, OT, nursing, nutrition, and social services.

Occupational Therapy Evaluation

Mary was evaluated by occupational therapy on the day of her admission to the transitional care unit. She was pleasant and cooperative, but needed to be redirected to remain focused. The evaluation revealed no deficits in cognition, perception, sensation, or hearing. She wears glasses at all times. Mary had some decreased AROM in both shoulders, possibly due to the osteoarthritis. Her AROM was at approximately 2/3 range for all shoulder motions. She had no range limitation in the elbows or wrist, but cannot make a full fist on the left hand without slight pain in the MCPs. She had a full grasp in the right hand, which is her dominant hand. Mary had (F−) strength in the shoulders, (F+) in the elbows and wrists and right hand. She had (F−/F) strength in the left hand. Her UE coordination was intact for both gross and fine motor. Mary had pain in the left hip only during motion. She had to adhere to total hip precautions and was allowed only partial weight-bearing on the affected extremity. Mary did not like to talk about the surgery and would not look at the incision. When the nurse came in to give her medication and check on or change the dressing, Mary would either turn and look the other way or close her eyes.

Mary had some slight edema in her left LE. She was at risk for skin breakdown because of the limited motion of her hip and her sleeping position at night. Her bed mobility was fair. She rolled in bed with moderate assistance, bracing herself for pain the whole time. She moved from supine to sit with moderate assistance. She seemed afraid to place any weight on her left leg and performed her transfers slowly and hesitantly. Mary used a standard walker for her transfers. She transferred from bed to wheelchair with the maximum assistance of one person. She tightly clung to the therapist the entire time and did little to help herself through the transfer. She transferred in a squat-pivot manner instead of a stand-pivot, which she should have been able to do. She performed toilet transfers at the same level of ability.

Mary was able to perform her upper body bathing and dressing independently. She refused to allow the male nursing assistants to help her and was even hesitant about the female care staff. She was not able to perform her lower body self-care due to her hip precautions. Mary states she was very scared to "pop it out" and have to go through "it" again. The occupational therapist attempted to explain the long-handled adaptive equipment to her but she declined until "the time is right for my leg."

Mary stated her goals are to go home as soon as she can and to care for herself and her home independently. She said she wants to walk without a cane and be able to get up and down stairs without pain. Mary said she is willing to work with occupational therapy as long as she does not have to use any "gadgets."

QUESTIONS

Goals/Treatment Plan

1. Write out a problem list for Mary.

2. Write out a list of Mary's strengths.

3. What long-term goals would you and Mary set for her occupational therapy treatment?

4. What would be appropriate short-term goals for Mary's OT treatment?

5. What do you anticipate to be some of the obstacles for Mary in reaching her goals?

6. What will be some of the difficulties for you as a therapist to help Mary reach her goals?

7. Write out a specific treatment plan for Mary including the frequency of OT sessions. Be prepared to explain why you decided to establish the plan you've devised.

Safety/Precautions

8. What are posterolateral total hip precautions?

9. Explain these in terms that will be easy for Mary to understand.

10. What devices will be needed for Mary to adhere to total hip precautions while toileting? While sleeping?

NOTES

Self-Care/Work/Leisure

11. How would you have Mary perform her ADLs given her limitations from total hip replacement?

12. What portion of the ADL routine do you anticipate will be most difficult for her to accomplish?

13. How might you adapt this portion of the ADL routine to maximize independence?

14. What do you think would be Mary's ability to prepare a meal? Support your answer with data.

15. What are some of Mary's social and leisure needs?

16. How could Mary's social and leisure needs be met on the unit?

Equipment/Adaptations

17. If Mary refuses to use the adaptive equipment, what alternatives could you offer Mary to help her reach her goals?

18. What questions would you ask her to determine what environmental adaptations might be needed for her transition safely back home?

19. What approach might you take to reintroduce the adaptive equipment to Mary to help her reach her goals?

Neuromusculoskeletal

20. What would you do to address Mary's neuromusculoskeletal status?

21. Mary says she'll participate in only one group in the unit. Which one do you think would be the most beneficial and why?

Psychosocial

22. How do you think Mary is dealing with her transitional care unit placement? What strategies is she using to cope with her change in health?

23. What feelings do you think Mary might have regarding her recent surgery and why?

24. How might the staff react to Mary's personality? Give two reactions that are positive and two that are not.

25. How can you prevent yourself from responding negatively to Mary?

26. What might be some psychological concerns for Mary when she leaves the transitional care unit?

Patient/Family Education

27. What educational information is essential for Mary? Why?

Situations

28. You enter Mary's room in the morning, and she has gotten a nursing assistant to do all her self-care for her. What might you say and/or do?

29. You enter Mary's room and find the nursing assistant partly finished with Mary's self-care. What would your reaction be at that time and why?

NOTES

30. Suppose you overhear Mary talking to her roommate about the therapists at the facility. Mary says that you are a "pain in the butt" for trying to make her use all those "crazy gadgets." What, if anything, do you do?

31. How would it make you feel to know that Mary is annoyed by your attempts to help her?

32. You are in the OT kitchen with Mary practicing making tea. You notice that Mary is not putting any weight on her left LE. "I don't want to take any chances," she says. How do you deal with this?

33. While transferring to the commode, Mary cries out in pain. She says it is her left hip and describes it as a burning pain that shoots down her leg. What do you do?

34. How would you document this incident? Where in the chart would you document it?

Discharge Planning

35. When would you begin discharge planning with Mary?

36. At what level of ability would Mary need to be to return home?

37. What role would her sister play in the discharge process? What role would Mary play?

38. How might Mary continue to work toward her goals once she leaves the unit?

39. Would you recommend continued OT for Mary at home? Why or why not?

40. If you did recommend OT at home, would you still do it if Mary told you she didn't want it?

41. If you didn't recommend OT at home, what would you want to have in place for Mary to function in her home safely?

NOTES

Chapter 14

Nellie:
Compression Fractures T12-L2

Nellie is an 84-year-old French-Canadian female with a diagnosis of compression fractures of the T12-L2 vertebrae, which she sustained from a fall. Nellie has a past medical history of osteoporosis, hypertension, insulin-dependent diabetes mellitus, peripheral neuropathy, legal blindness, and status post right hip fracture with open reduction internal fixation (ORIF) last year, also as the result of a fall.

Nellie has been able to continue living in the community with the support of her daughters. She is able to sponge bathe and dress herself sitting at a chair by the bathroom sink; she does not use the shower or tub. Once a week, her daughter Connie, 66, comes from across town to wash and set her hair for her. Nellie's family does all of the housekeeping and cooking for her. Sally comes once a week and does her mother's laundry and cleans the house thoroughly. Millie comes every morning and makes her mother breakfast and gives her insulin and her other medications. Millie will then make Nellie a light lunch and put it in the refrigerator for her mother to have when she is hungry. Millie then comes back again in the evening and brings her mother some supper. Sometimes, Millie will bring her own meal downstairs and eat with her mother.

Prior to her hospitalization, Nellie had been living in a three-family home, which she owns in a rural area. Nellie lives alone on the first floor and her youngest daughter, Sally, 62, lives on the second floor with her husband, Karl. On the third floor lives Nellie's oldest daughter, Millie, 68, who is recently widowed. Nellie is from Quebec and has been living in this country since she was in her 40s. Nellie speaks and reads English well, although her primary language is French.

Nellie does not drive. Her daughters do all of her shopping and outside errands. They also take turns bringing her to any appointments she has with physicians. Nellie's son-in-law Karl takes out her trash and does all the repairs necessary on the house himself or makes arrangements to hire someone to do what he cannot. Karl takes care of the yard and pays all of Nellie's bills for her.

Nellie has one son, Tom, who lives in Ontario. He calls her every week, but she sees him only twice a year. Nellie has never worked outside the home. She has been widowed for the last 12 years. She and her husband married young and would have been married almost 55 years when he died. She misses him terribly. Since his death, Nellie's health has been deteriorating. She is much less active without her life-long partner and tends to lean on her daughters even more. She had enjoyed traveling, but had stopped all of that after her husband died. Nellie is also limited by her vision, which has gotten progressively worse. This makes her feel even more isolated from non-family members.

Nellie had been ambulating with a standard walker. She is not able to climb stairs without someone's assistance. Her last fall, which resulted in a fractured hip, was due to tripping on the bathroom throw rug. The fall that led to this hospitalization occurred when Nellie was sitting at the edge of the bed. Because of the peripheral neuropathy in her bilateral lower extremities, she says she thought her feet were securely on the floor, but they were not. She slipped off the edge of the bed and landed on her back. This resulted in the compression fractures of her low back at T12-L2.

Nellie has been admitted to the transitional care unit from the acute wing of the hospital. The plan is for her to be here for 2 weeks and then possibly go to a nursing and rehabilitation center if more therapy and/or nursing care is required. Nellie believes the plan is for her to return home. Her daughters want the same thing, but are concerned for their mother's safety since she's fallen twice in the last year. Nellie will receive nursing, PT, OT, social service, recreational, and nutrition services while at the transitional care unit.

Occupational Therapy Evaluation

Upon evaluation, Nellie exhibits a decrease in short-term memory and difficulty problem-solving new information. She has decreased sensation (light/deep touch, hot/cold) in her bilateral upper extremities. The PT evaluation revealed almost absent sensation in her feet. Nellie has impugned stereognosis recognizing only two out of four items placed in her hand. Her proprioception and kinesthesia are intact. As stated, she is legally blind and can see only shapes and lights. Her hearing is intact as are her language skills. She has AROM WFL in her UEs. She has F+ strength overall and her coordination is also WFL. Her fine-motor ability is limited by her vision (eye-hand coordination). She is left-hand dominant.

Nellie has pain in her low back and wears a back binder for protection. She is unable to bend to reach her LE and cannot rotate or laterally flex her trunk. She has no edema or skin changes.

She is able to perform all bed mobility and transfers with minimum to moderate assistance depending on her level of fatigue and pain. Shower transfers are not assessed, as Nellie did not perform them prior to admission. Nellie is using the standard walker she brought from home for all mobility.

Nellie is able to sponge bathe her upper body and perineal area. She is dependent for LE, back, and buttock bathing. She states she uses a long-handled sponge at home and can bathe herself with minimum assistance. She is able to dress her upper body independently but requires total assistance for donning pants and underpants over her feet. Nellie is able to pull up garments with minimum assistance. She is dependent for donning and doffing socks and can put on shoes independently because she wears only slippers. Nellie said she wears shoes only to her doctor's appointments.

Nellie understands that the reason for her therapy is to be able to care for herself again. Her goals for OT are to dress and bathe herself again. Nellie says she doesn't want to ask her daughters to have to do any more for her than they already do.

QUESTIONS

Goals/Treatment Plan

1. Write out a problem list for Nellie.

2. What functional limitations would you not address with Nellie? Why?

3. What are Nellie's strengths?

4. What short- and long-term goals would you and Nellie set for her occupational therapy treatment?

5. What obstacles do you see for Nellie as she works toward her goals?

6. What goals do you think Nellie's family have in mind for her?

7. How do you think the family's goals will affect Nellie's goals? Why?

8. Write out a specific treatment plan for Nellie including frequency.

9. Would you involve Nellie in any of the groups on the unit? If so, which ones?

Safety/Precautions

10. What are some safety issues that might arise for Nellie?

11. What are ways in which OT and the other team members might work with Nellie to reduce her safety risk?

NOTES

12. What suggestions might you give the family to help keep Nellie safe?

13. What are the precautions following compression fractures?

Self-Care/Work/Leisure

14. How would you set up Nellie's materials for an ADL treatment?

15. What home management skills would you address with Nellie?

Equipment/Adaptations

16. What adaptive equipment would Nellie need to help her achieve her goals with OT?

17. What difficulties might Nellie encounter in trying to use the adaptive equipment?

18. Given that her family helps her with most tasks, do you think it is worth it to train Nellie to use the adaptive equipment?

Neuromusculoskeletal

19. What would you do to address Nellie's back pain? Explain.

20. What would you do to address Nellie's strength deficits?

21. What would you do to address Nellie's sensation deficits?

22. What is the definition of legally blind? What strategies would you use to help Nellie compensate for this deficit?

Cognition/Perception

23. Nellie's short-term memory is not reliable. She keeps confusing staff members and feels embarrassed about it. What can be done to help her with this?

Psychosocial

24. What psychological impact might the hospitalization have on Nellie?

25. What psychological impact might the hospitalization have on Nellie's family?

26. What are some ways to support Nellie and her family through the rehabilitation process?

Patient/Family Education

27. Which family member would you teach to assist Nellie with her ADLs?

28. Describe how you would teach that person to assist with donning and doffing the back brace.

29. Explain how you would educate Nellie to prevent further falls.

29a. Explain how you would educate Nellie's family to prevent further falls.

30. What factors may interfere with the educational portion of OT treatment?

31. How would you overcome this?

NOTES

Situations

32. Nellie is unable to perform lower body ADLs even with adaptive equipment because of pain and poor eyesight. What alternatives might be available for her to allow greater independence in daily personal care?

33. Nellie tells you that the adaptive equipment is difficult to use and that when she gets home she will most likely just wear slippers with no socks, a dress, and no underwear. What is your response?

34. Nellie reaches her initial ADL goals after only a few days at the TCU. Would you discharge her from OT at that time? Why?

35. Suppose Nellie's daughter Millie becomes ill while Nellie is at the TCU and will no longer be able to provide help to her mother as before. How will this change the course of Nellie's hospital stay? Explain.

36. Suppose Nellie's daughter Sally becomes ill while Nellie is at the TCU and will no longer be able to provide help to her mother as before. How will this change the course of Nellie's hospital stay? Explain.

37. You perform the Kohlman Evaluation of Living Skills (KELS) with Nellie and she scores as follows: needs assistance in all areas except telephoning and knowledge of emergency numbers. How do you use this information?

38. The physical therapist doesn't think Nellie is safe to go home. The social worker feels she is safe to return to her prior living arrangement. Who do you agree with and why?

39. Would you respond differently to the question above if different professionals were involved, if, for example, the physiatrist were in the place of the social worker and the nurse were in the place of the PT?

40. One of Nellie's daughters wants her to move in with her instead of living alone. Nellie asks your advice. What do you say?

41. If you were Nellie, what would be the positives and negatives of moving in with one of your daughters?

Discharge Planning

42. When would you feel Nellie would be ready to go home? How would you know?

43. How might you help Nellie to best prepare for the transition back home?

44. What type of services, if any, would you recommend for Nellie at home?

45. How would you arrange for those services in your own community? State two resources that are available.

46. Would you recommend OT for Nellie at home? Why and for what?

47. If Nellie and her family felt that it was not safe for her to return home, what might be some of their placement options?

48. Which of those options do you think would be best for Nellie and why?

Chapter 15

Oscar:
Pneumonia,
Chronic Obstructive Pulmonary Disease

Oscar is a 91-year-old Caucasian man who has been living with his granddaughter prior to his hospitalization. He was diagnosed with chronic obstructive pulmonary disease 17 years ago and had a two-pack-a-day smoking habit for 45 years. Additional diagnoses include hearing loss, spinal stenosis L-4 and L-5, and congestive heart failure (CHF). Oscar quit smoking 16 years ago and had been functioning without supplemental oxygen prior to the admission to the transitional care unit. He was initially hospitalized 4 weeks ago at the acute care hospital with a diagnosis of pneumonia. He was on IV antibiotics and due to the CHF and his age, took a long time to recover. He lost 10 pounds and became deconditioned at the hospital due to the prolonged bedrest.

Prior to his hospitalization, Oscar was functioning at a moderate assistance level for his bathing and dressing, and was dependent for all meals, even a light breakfast of toast, coffee, and cereal. Oscar lives with his granddaughter Stacey, who takes care of all home management tasks, such as laundry, meal preparation, and grocery and clothes shopping. Stacey is a single mother with two teenaged sons. She works part-time as a salesperson in a retail clothing shop. Stacey and Oscar live in his home, which is a ranch house that is paid off. Stacey will keep the house when Oscar dies. Oscar's room is on the main floor, and her sons have a room in the finished basement. There are four steps to enter the home. Oscar has a TV in his room, and the bathroom is off the hall about 10 feet from his room.

Oscar is long retired from his job as a sales representative for a rug manufacturer. He no longer goes out of the house and does not have contact with anyone except Stacey and his two great-grandsons. Oscar and his great-grandsons don't spend much time together. He is a cantankerous man who is used to having his needs met by his granddaughter. He keeps to himself, enjoys playing the lottery, and spends his days watching TV. His favorite shows are police shows and Bowling for Dollars.

Discharge plans are for Oscar to return to his prior living arrangement. He is being seen by occupational therapy, physical therapy, and nursing. He was admitted to the transitional care unit of the acute care hospital. His granddaughter calls weekly but doesn't visit. Oscar's goals are to return to his home. He does not wish to be more independent than he previously was. Stacey expresses her goals that Oscar be more independent in his ADLs.

Occupational Therapy Evaluation

Occupational therapy evaluated Oscar on the day of admission. He is quite fatigued after the transfer from the hospital unit and the nursing admission, but policy dictates that the evaluation be completed on the day of admission. He appears alert but very tired. He wears glasses, has dentures, and is hard of hearing. He owns a hearing aid, but hasn't worn it in many years. He turns on the TV loudly and can hear when speech is slow and clear. Perception and sensation appear intact upon observation. Oscar is alert and oriented to self and place, but not time. He is unable to explain why he is in the SNF or where he was prior to this. He remembers his granddaughter and events from the past, but shows poor recall for recent events. His AROM is WFL for his age with shoulder weakness of 4/5 bilaterally. He demonstrates intact coordination and hand dexterity. He is right-handed. Oscar tolerates less than 5 minutes of low-endurance activities. He is currently on oxygen via nasal canula at 2 liters for rest and 3 liters for activity.

Oscar requires moderate assistance for transfers in and out of bed due to leg weakness. He is able to roll in bed holding onto the siderails. He currently requires a wheelchair for distances and is dependent for wheelchair mobility. Oscar ambulates in his room with a walker and moderate assistance.

Oscar is too weak to assess showering, and his ADL status is limited to washing his hands and face while sitting in bed. He has only worn hospital gowns, but the expectation is that he will be maximum assist with dressing due to his deconditioned status.

Oscar is tired and grouchy at the time of the evaluation and anxious to get some rest. He states that he wants to be "like I was before this damned pneumonia!" and wants to return to his granddaughter's home. He is in a double room in the transitional care unit.

QUESTIONS

Goals/Treatment Plan

1. What do you see as Oscar's strengths and weaknesses?

2. What did Oscar state as his goals for his rehab stay? Based on the occupational therapy evaluation, do you think Oscar can do more for himself than he was previously doing? If so, how will you deal with this during treatment?

3. Write a treatment plan for Oscar, making sure it reflects Oscar's goals.

4. How do you think Oscar's age might affect his rehabilitation program?

Safety/Precautions

5. What precautions are important to remember when working with someone who needs oxygen?

6. What safety issues must you instruct Oscar on in relation to his oxygen?

Self-Care/Work/Leisure

7. Oscar was very tired on the day of the OT evaluation, but is now feeling somewhat more energetic. How will you approach the task of ADL training with him? (What tasks will you work on first, second, etc.?) How will you grade the activities?

8. Oscar requires oxygen at 3 liters during bathing and dressing. Is it safe for him to shower with oxygen? How will you address this issue during his shower?

9. Oscar gets very short of breath with minimal exertion. During his shower, he begins to hyperventilate. What techniques would you teach him to use during this activity? How would you teach him?

10. Oscar tells you that his granddaughter usually gives him a shower twice a week and he really doesn't want to do it himself. You feel that he is capable of being at least moderate to minimum assist in showering with equipment. How do you handle this situation?

11. While working on dressing skills, Oscar is bending over to put on his pants. He is struggling with his pants, and you see his face becoming very red. Why do you think Oscar's face is getting red, and what should you do in this situation? How would you educate Oscar as to the reason this happened, and how would you prevent it from happening next time?

12. After 1 week on the TCU, Oscar is still having difficulty getting in and out of bed with the head of the hospital bed down flat. What activities could you do to address this deficit that would differentiate your treatment from the physical therapy treatment?

NOTES

13. Oscar is taken to the OT kitchen to do a light meal preparation (toast, coffee, and cereal). He is using a walker now. In training him to use the walker safely in the kitchen, how do you instruct him in hand placement when reaching? How do you instruct him to carry items (he has no walker basket) from the counter/refrigerator to the table, which is about 4 feet away?

14. During a treatment session, Oscar mentions that he used to have a beautiful garden in his own home. You ask some questions and find out that he also loved houseplants and had a beautiful collection a long time ago. Knowing how Oscar spent his leisure time prior to his TCU admission, would you address this leisure issue? If so, how?

Equipment/Adaptations

15. What types of adaptive equipment would you expect Oscar to need to accomplish the goals set for him? How much would this equipment cost? Which ones, if any, are covered by Medicare?

16. How will you recommend that Oscar's environment be adapted for his COPD?

17. How should Oscar's ADL routine be adapted to maximize his abilities?

Neuromusculoskeletal

18. Oscar is deconditioned due to his COPD and hospitalization. What type of conditioning program would you set up for him? How would you set up goals that differentiate occupational therapy from physical therapy in this area?

19. Can you identify some functional or purposeful treatment activities that will address Oscar's deconditioned status?

20. Using the activities from the question above, how can they be graded?

21. You know from the team meeting that the physical therapist is working on balance activities with Oscar. How can you incorporate this into your treatment activities?

Cognition/Perception

22. During the evaluation, Oscar showed some memory problems. How would you formally assess this? What assessment would you use and why? Does this assessment give you information related to his functional abilities?

23. Given Oscar's memory problem, how would you ensure carryover of your teaching of new information?

Psychosocial

24. Oscar has told you on several occasions that he is old and not afraid to die, that he would rather die than go to a nursing home. However, during the second week, he is still grouchy and not very motivated during treatment. How would you deal with this behavior?

25. Oscar likes to make sexual remarks to the female staff. Why do you think he is doing this, and how do you handle it when he makes them to you during a bathing activity?

Situations

26. Oscar's granddaughter has told you that she would like him to be more independent in bathing, dressing, and simple meal preparation or she won't take him home. She doesn't want to tell Oscar herself though and is depending on the team at the TCU to do this. How should you and the team handle this situation?

NOTES

27. Oscar tells you at the beginning of a treatment session that he wants you to walk him today, like his other therapist does. He says that he is more concerned about his walking than anything else. Can you think of a way to incorporate his request into a treatment session that will be different from physical therapy, but still be purposeful and meaningful?

28. How would you characterize Stacey and Oscar's relationship? Are there aspects of it that might beg help or hindrance in your treatment of Oscar?

Patient/Family Education

29. Oscar will need to go home with oxygen. What is necessary to educate Oscar and Stacey about? Do you include her teenaged sons in the education as well?

30. What techniques that you taught Oscar are important for Stacey to be taught?

31. Stacey is upset that Oscar is not getting better fast enough. She states that she won't take him home unless he is independent in his ADLs and can get himself his own breakfast. She has brought several of the certified nursing assistants to tears with her yelling. A family-team meeting is arranged to discuss Oscar's treatment plan, goals, current status, and discharge plans. You feel Oscar is progressing well, but that by discharge he will still not be independent in his ADLs due to his severely deconditioned status. You expect Oscar to need minimum assist with showering to wash his back, hair, and lower legs, setup for dressing using adaptive equipment, but dependent with his shoes and socks. As for making breakfast, you don't feel he is safe with hot liquids at the walker level, but could manage making toast and cereal with some minimal modifications to give him easy access to the materials. You also feel that Oscar is intimidated by his granddaughter and will not ask her for assistance. How will you present your impressions of Oscar at the meeting so that Stacey doesn't get defensive and will agree with the discharge plan of his returning home at the current level?

32. Oscar talks about his granddaughter sometimes not getting his dinner ready until 9 P.M. or not washing him until late in the day. What do you do with this information?

Discharge Planning

33. Given Oscar's situation in Question 31, if Oscar returns to his home at discharge, what services, if any would you recommend upon his discharge to his home?

NOTES

Part V

Skilled Nursing Facility

Chapter 16

Paula:
Parkinson's Disease

Paula is a 76-year-old Caucasian female with a diagnosis of Parkinson's disease and secondary diagnoses of cataracts and hypertension. Paula is retired from her job as a professor of history at an area college. Prior to her admission to the skilled nursing facility, Paula was living at home with her husband, Dave, and had been receiving home care services for bathing, dressing, laundry, and light housekeeping 7 days a week. Paula and Dave both receive Meals on Wheels 5 days a week. The home-care agency had to cut back on the services they were providing due to changes in Medicare reimbursement, and this left a hole in Paula's ability to remain at home with her aging husband, who is unable to care for her and the home. She was admitted to the skilled nursing facility in the same town she and her husband have lived in for 45 years.

Although retired as a history professor, Paula kept up with colleagues at the college where she taught, maintained an office at the college (although she rarely went in), and had contact with former students and colleagues through the Internet. She spent much of her time at the computer in her home office. She continued to review manuscripts for a publishing company as well as a professional journal.

Paula and Dave have one daughter, but she lives far away and cannot be a part of their daily support services. She is in touch with her parents every few days by phone and visits every other month. Their daughter works and has two small children of her own.

Paula is a strong-willed and independent person who does not like being in the skilled nursing facility, but is resigned to it. She did explore assisted-living facilities, but she and her husband could not afford this option. She misses her husband, the contact via Internet with her colleagues, and her own home and the independence it afforded her.

Paula was admitted onto the skilled nursing unit for long-term care. All residents upon admission are screened by occupational and physical therapy. Minimum Data Sets (MDS) are completed with each team member completing the appropriate section and a team meeting is set within 7 days to discuss the treatment plan and goals.

Paula was screened by occupational therapy and a subsequent occupational therapy evaluation was requested to gather more data on her functional skills in bathing, dressing, feeding, cognition, and psychosocial status.

Occupational Therapy Evaluation

Paula demonstrates intact cognition, sensation, perception, and hearing, but has decreased visual acuity due to cataracts.

Her UE AROM is WFL bilaterally, muscle strength is 4/5 in the shoulder muscles on both sides, and 4+/5 in the remainder of her UEs, with her right side being her dominant side. She demonstrates very poor trunk control, however, and cannot sit unsupported for greater than 5 minutes before she begins to slide down and lean to the left in the chair. She demonstrates the ability to sit unsupported for about 30 seconds before slouching and lateral trunk flexion to the left begins. Her head is laterally flexed to the left as well. She has decreased neck ROM both passive and active, with only about 1/3 of full head rotation present. She has decreased gross- and fine-motor coordination in both UEs. Her handwriting is illegible, and her movements are slow. There are intention tremors in both her UEs of a mild type, but the tremor increases with effortful activity and makes it difficult for her to use her right arm during functional activities. She has moderate tone in her LEs, with the left leg having increased tremor and spasticity with effortful movement and at rest. This leg flexes at the knee and hip during any activity in sitting leading to poor sitting balance. The right leg has mildly increased tremor, but does not interfere with function. Paula's trunk is rigid and moves as if a log with no dissociation between her upper and lower trunk.

She ambulates with a rolling walker, but does not like to use it, and ambulates by holding onto the furniture to get to the bed or chair. At home, she experienced frequent falls and had taken to wearing kneepads to protect herself from the inevitable falls. When moved from stand to sit, she gets near the chair or bed and just flops down any old way, sometimes coming close to missing altogether. Bed mobility is independent but effortful. She is able to roll side to side using the bedrails; she uses the controls of the hospital bed to raise the head of the bed to assist in sitting up.

She has difficulty bathing at the sink. She sits on the toilet to sponge bathe her upper body, but due to her poor sitting balance, she slides off the toilet onto the floor. She is unable to bend over and wash her lower torso, and dresses her upper body slowly, requiring moderate assistance with her lower body. She has difficulty with buttons, but can eventually get them all done. She is dependent for her shoes and stockings. She is able to feed herself, but her hands shake when lifting glasses, mugs, and her silverware. It takes her a very long time to eat and to cut up her food. Her swallowing is intact, but drooling does occur during activities that require a lot of effort.

She is short-tempered with the staff, although this is not her usual personality. She states she doesn't want to participate in the activity program and says the groups are "boring" and for the "mentally challenged." She doesn't understand what occupational therapy is and states she "already has an occupation." She misses her husband, who is still living in their home, and the contact with her academic colleagues and students.

Paula wants more than anything to be able to bring her computer in and have Internet access so she can stay "mentally with it." She shares a room with another resident who loves to watch TV most of the day. Her roommate leaves the TV on even when she isn't there and doesn't want anyone to turn it off. Paula's goals also include independence in daily bathing and dressing and to eat in the dining room.

QUESTIONS

Goals/Treatment Plan

1. Paula doesn't have a clear understanding of the role of occupational therapy. How would you explain your role to her so that she would be invested in her occupational therapy program?

2. Write a problem list for Paula.

3. Write long- and short-term goals for Paula.

4. List the treatment activities that you will use with Paula.

5. What part of the treatment plan is appropriate for a COTA to do?

6. What other team members would you consult and collaborate with?

Safety/Precautions

7. What are some of the safety concerns for Paula? How would you prioritize these?

8. Besides Paula's Parkinson's disease, which other diagnoses could pose safety issues for her and why?

9. How will you go about working with Paula on these issues?

10. What equipment might you recommend?

Notes

Self-Care/Work/Leisure

11. What would you identify as Paula's major problem in the work/leisure area?

12. What would you do to address this problem?

13. In what way might you enlist the support of Paula's husband around her work/leisure activities?

14. What would you identify as the major obstacle(s) for Paula in being independent in bathing, dressing, and feeding?

15. How would you address this/these in treatment?

16. How would you address Paula's difficulty at mealtime?

17. How would you educate other staff about your mealtime recommendations?

Equipment/Adaptations

18. What type of adaptive equipment would you use with Paula to assist with bathing, dressing, and feeding?

19. How would you teach Paula to use the adaptive equipment recommended?

20. What type of seating equipment would you use to position Paula properly? Remember, customized wheelchairs are not usually paid for when in an SNF.

Neuromusculoskeletal

21. What are Paula's deficits in her UEs?

22. How would these deficits affect her functionally throughout her day?

23. What type of treatment activities would you use to address Paula's musculoskeletal status?

24. Parkinson's disease is characterized by rigidity and tremors. How would you address these as they are seen in Paula?

25. Would an exercise program be beneficial for Paula? Please explain your answer.

Psychosocial

26. What are the psychosocial issues that need addressing with Paula?

27. How would you address these issues in your treatment sessions?

28. What other individuals might you enlist to help in this area? What types of groups might be meaningful to Paula?

Patient/Family Education

29. Given that Parkinson's disease is a progressive neurological disease, how would you teach Paula about the functional import of the disease?

30. Explain to Paula the importance of using the rolling walker during functional activities.

NOTES

Situations

31. At the team meeting, Paula is identified by the dietician as a high risk for aspiration and wants to start her on a ground diet. You feel that Paula needs dysphagia treatment before changing her diet. How do you address this issue in the team meeting?

32. The CNAs see Paula as a very difficult resident. She requires a lot of their time at meals and for ADLs because she is so slow. They want to do everything for her so they can get on to their next resident, but Paula gets angry at them because she wants to remain as independent as possible and do as much for herself as she is able. How do you address this issue with the CNAs who care for Paula daily?

Discharge Planning

33. Paula has refused to participate in treatment for the past week, stating she just doesn't feel like doing anything. What are some of the possible reasons for this, and what would you do?

34. How would you ensure that gains made during your OT treatments are maintained once Paula is discharged from therapy?

NOTES

Chapter 17

Quinn: Dementia

Quinn is a 77-year-old Caucasian man with a diagnosis of dementia. Quinn has a past medical history of congestive heart failure, hypertension, depression, and gout. Quinn has been a resident at the nursing home for the last 2 years. He resides on the long-term care wing of the facility. It is the family's plan that Quinn remain at the nursing home indefinitely.

Quinn's wife, Dorothea, visits on Wednesdays and Fridays. She takes him outside onto the patio and reads him letters from their grandchildren. When she has no family news, she reads him the newspaper or the church bulletin. Dorothea wants Quinn to remain as mentally capable as possible. It is obvious that there is a strong bond between them. Dorothea holds Quinn's hand for her entire visit. She attends all of his care plan meetings and frequently speaks as an advocate on his behalf.

Quinn participates minimally in the facility's activities. If someone wheels him into the day room, he'll listen to the radio or watch the entertainers. Quinn speaks only if spoken to or if he needs something. He uses simple sentences and often answers incorrectly when asked simple questions. Quinn recognizes Dorothea, but sometimes confuses his daughters and grandchildren. He cannot recall the names of staff members, but does smile when he sees someone he recognizes.

The nurse, who realized Quinn is now requiring more assistance from the nursing assistants at meals, has referred him to occupational therapy. Quinn had been eating in the main dining room for lunch and dinner, but now has to eat in the day room on the unit because he requires assistance with his meals. Such one-on-one assistance is not available in the main dining room.

Upon speaking to the nurse and his primary nursing assistant, it becomes clear that Quinn has been requiring more help with his meals over the last 3 to 4 weeks. He had required only setup with his meals in the past. Reportedly, he now needs to be fed. Quinn has been dependent for his ADLs since he arrived at the facility and is non-ambulatory. The facility staff feels that Quinn is more cognitively impaired than he appears.

Because Quinn is not newly admitted to the facility, it is the policy of the occupational therapy department to use a specialized feeding evaluation for long-term residents. A feeding evaluation is performed with Quinn.

Occupational Therapy Evaluation

Quinn is sitting in a wheelchair that his family purchased for him (Figure 17-1). His leg rests are elevated to prevent LE edema. The wheelchair that Quinn sits in has a reclining back, and he is leaning back at approximately a 35° angle. His pelvis is tilted posteriorly, his head is jutting forward, and his cervical spine is in a kyphotic posture.

Quinn has AROM WNL for his UEs through slightly less flexion of the shoulders secondary to the kyphosis. His strength is G−/F+ and his gross-motor control is WFL. His fine-motor coordination is impaired but could not be formally assessed due to his cognitive status. His sensation appears intact for both UEs but could not be formally assessed either. He is right-hand dominant.

Cognitively, Quinn displays short- and long-term memory deficits and a decrease in executive functions. He is able to follow some verbal commands accompanied by visual cues, such as "shake my hand." He is unable to learn new information, but performs automatic responses without prompting. He has an attention span of approximately 5 minutes. He is oriented to self only. Quinn is on a regular diet.

Quinn requires setup for his meal. He is unable to identify and locate the various utensils used during his meal. However, he is able to demonstrate holding a spoon and a fork correctly once it is properly placed in his

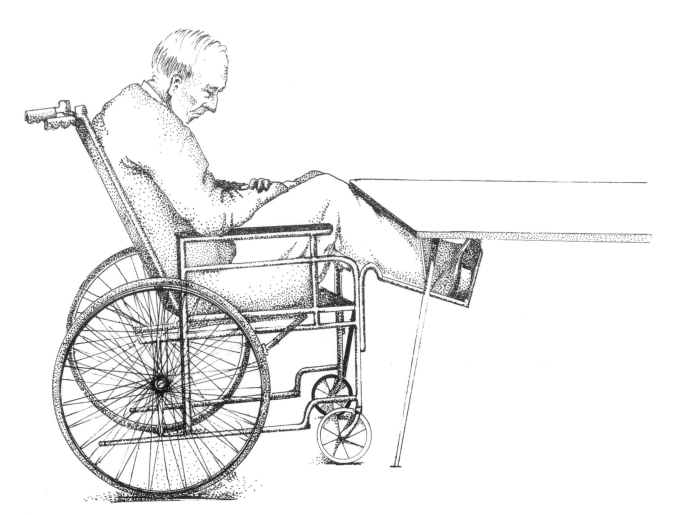

Figure 17-1.

hand. Quinn has much difficulty scooping the food onto the spoon. He is unable to successfully pierce food with a fork six out of 10 tries. Quinn also has difficulty not dropping the food once he has successfully gotten it onto his utensil. While bringing it to his mouth, many pieces fall into his lap. Quinn then puts the fork or spoon down and picks the pieces up with his fingers. He gets the pieces of food into his mouth every time.

Quinn is able to eat a piece of buttered bread independently once it is placed in his hand. Quinn is also able to hold a cup independently, again, only after it is placed in his hand. He is only able to drink half of his liquid because he cannot extend his neck from the flexed position to tip the remainder of the liquid out of the glass. He is able to continue drinking once given a straw. However, he neglects to use the straw the next time the cup is placed in his hand. He does not finish his drink without assistance. Quinn uses his napkin spontaneously once placed in his hand.

Quinn is unable to state his goals for occupational therapy. He does not appear to understand the purpose of occupational therapy. The purpose and projected outcome of occupational therapy is explained to his wife. She repeats her own goal of having her husband be able to eat in the dining room at meals. She agrees for OT services to begin.

QUESTIONS

Goals/Treatment Plan

1. Write out a problem list for Quinn.

2. What strengths do you see that Quinn has to help him achieve his goals?

NOTES

3. What short-term goals would you set for Quinn to help reach the long-term goal of eating in the main dining room?

4. What obstacles do you see for Quinn in reaching his goals?

5. Write out a specific treatment plan for Quinn including frequency and duration.

Safety/Precautions

6. You adjust Quinn's wheelchair so he sits upright at a 90° angle. He slowly begins to slip out of his chair. Explain what you do in this situation.

7. Make a list of all the possible complications Quinn might have because of his position in the wheelchair.

Self-Care/Work/Leisure

8. Describe a single OT treatment session with Quinn, focusing on increasing independence at meals.

9. What techniques might you use to facilitate the skills needed to improve his self-feeding abilities?

Equipment/Adaptations

10. What type of environmental adaptations need to be made for Quinn to allow him to feed himself more independently?

11. What type of adaptive equipment might Quinn need to enable him to be independent in self-feeding? How does food texture influence self-feeding? Do you think Quinn needs a change in textures?

12. Explain how you would involve the dietary and nursing staff in this process.

12a. Using Figure 17-1, describe what is correct and incorrect with Quinn's wheelchair positioning.

Neuromusculoskeletal

13. What can be done to treat Quinn's decrease in fine-motor coordination?

Cognition/Perception

14. What can be done to treat Quinn's cognitive deficits? What compensatory strategies will you use for the cognitive deficits you cannot treat?

Psychosocial

15. What psychological impact do you think being fed may have on Quinn?

16. What impact do you think it may have on his wife? What type of support do you think might benefit Dorothea as Quinn's condition progresses? What other disciplines might you refer Dorothea to?

Patient/Family Education

17. Write out how you would explain Quinn's abilities to his wife.

Situations

18. You have made changes in Quinn's mealtime routine and want other staff to follow through with your interventions. Name all the staff who are involved and what type of teaching you must do to ensure the program carryover that you want.

NOTES

19. Quinn becomes agitated when you try to rearrange his plate to facilitate independence. He refuses to eat after you have intervened. What do you do?

20. Dorothea wants to see how her husband is doing in therapy. She asks what can she do to help promote independence. What do you tell her?

21. Dorothea decides to visit Quinn during the day at lunch. She wants him to sit on the patio with her. There is no table out there. What adaptations would you need to make to enable Quinn to eat his lunch on the patio with Dorothea?

22. You arrive at the facility early and go in to see how Quinn is doing with his breakfast. You see his nursing assistant feeding him oatmeal. What do you do?

23. This same scenario occurs several days in a row. Why might be some of the reasons as to why the nursing assistants keep feeding him day after day?

24. How would you deal with staff enabling Quinn's dependence at meals?

Discharge Planning

25. When you decide to discharge Quinn from OT services, what do you need to have in place to ensure he would be able to maintain his current level of independence?

26. How could you monitor Quinn to see that he did not decline again to being fed at meals?

NOTES

Chapter 18

Rob:
Blindness,
Non-Insulin-Dependent Diabetes Mellitus

Rob is an 83-year-old Caucasian man with a diagnosis of glaucoma, non-insulin dependent diabetes mellitus, gout, and hypertension. He is blind due to the glaucoma. He has been living in a skilled nursing facility for 1 month and has been having a difficult time adjusting to the new environment.

Prior to his admission to the skilled nursing facility, he had been living alone in his own house with services of a home health aide (HHA), homemaker, Meals on Wheels, and weekly nursing visits to monitor his insulin levels and blood pressure. He has been widowed for 6 years. A neighbor was also helping him with meals on the weekends and errands, as well with companionship. However, she was hospitalized herself and is no longer able to assist Rob, given that her assistance was one of the reasons Rob had been able to stay at home so long. Rob has a son, but they are not close and he is not available to help; therefore, placement was sought in a nearby skilled nursing facility.

Rob is a retired factory foreman. He has been retired for 18 years and has lived on Social Security and a small pension plan. Rob lost his vision gradually due to glaucoma. He knows his way around his home and had been able to remain there because of the services and the familiar environment. Rob is fiercely independent and is not happy about having to go into a skilled nursing facility. He uses talking books and listens to the TV. He enjoys going out for walks with his HHA in the nice weather.

In the skilled nursing facility, Rob has been having a difficult time adjusting to the loss of independence and to the institutional routines. A referral was made to OT by Rob's physician to assess his ability to be more independent in ADLs, mobility around the facility, and to work on leisure skills. He is being seen only by occupational therapy.

Occupational Therapy Evaluation

Rob has no observable deficits in his cognition or hearing. Sensation is impaired in his hands for hot/cold, sharp/dull, and light touch. He is blind due to the glaucoma, but can detect shadows and differences in light levels (bright light versus low light). He can recognize familiar people by their footsteps and voices.

Rob's AROM is WFL for his age with strength at the 4/5 bilaterally. He suffers from frequent onsets of gout in his left great toe which are extremely painful and leave him unable to get around without a wheelchair. He is left-handed and has no significant deficits in gross-motor coordination, but due to the sensory deficits in his hands, he has difficulty manipulating small objects, including buttons, pant zippers, and shoelaces. Except when he is experiencing an episode of gout, he does not have any pain.

Rob is able to move from supine to sit, sit to supine, and from sit to stand independently. He ambulates without any assistive device, but bumps into objects in his room and the environment outside his room. He is unable to find his own room if he is in the hallway. He spends a lot of time standing in the doorway to his room and talks to people who come by, but he is very reluctant to leave the room itself. Rob shares his room with one other gentleman who has Alzheimer's disease.

Rob requires setup for washing at the sink in the bathroom and for dressing because he has trouble finding his supplies and clothing. The staff never put things back in the same place. He has difficulty with the buttons on his shirts and with the zipper on his pants, and needs someone to tie his shoelaces for him.

Rob eats in the main dining room of the facility at a table with three other residents, where he enjoys the socialization. Rob can feed himself if someone cuts up the food and opens the containers and milk cartons. However, he doesn't know what the meal is until he starts to eat it and is not sure when he has eaten all the food on his plate. He knocks his glass over often and has difficulty locating his coffee cup on the table. He finds meals to be a frustrating experience and gets embarrassed by his clumsiness. The other people at his table try to help him as much as they can.

He alternates between feeling frustrated and depressed. He misses his independence and feels that he would be better in his own home, where he knows where everything is, but his son has put the house on the market and does not want him to go back home. When questioned about his interests, he says that "being blind took care of that." He used to fish, was in a bowling league with his wife, and enjoyed classical music. Now all he does is listen to the TV and occasionally the talking books.

Rob is open to OT and has stated that his goals are to be able to "do more for myself." When questioned further, he stated that his dignity is most important to him and he wanted to be able to bathe and dress himself, and to eat his meals without all the frustrations. He will be seen five times a week. His insurance is Medicare Part A.

QUESTIONS

Goals/Treatment Plan

1. What special considerations should you have when working with someone who is blind?

2. What are Rob's strengths and deficits?

3. Write long- and short-term goals for Rob.

4. If you were the OTR, what portions of the treatment plan would you have the COTA complete, and how would you monitor Rob's progress in these areas?

5. If you were the COTA, how would you collaborate with the OTR on this case?

6. How do you think Rob's psychological status will impact his motivation during therapy? How can you help to motivate him?

Safety/Precautions

7. Do you think that Rob is safe in his current environment? If not, what would you change and how? If yes, why do you think he is safe?

Self-Care/Work/Leisure

8. Please write your treatment activities for 1 week's worth of treatment to work on Rob's bathing and dressing deficits.

9. Mealtime is a very stressful time for Rob. What recommendations would you make to increase his independence and reduce his anxiety at meals?

10. How would you go about implementing your recommendations and getting the cooperation of the dining room staff (mostly CNAs and diet technicians)?

11. When Rob is not engaged in therapy, he spends his time standing in the doorway to his room chatting with staff, residents, and family members or in his room listening to TV. He has indicated that he wishes he could do something else with his time as he gets bored. He states that he isn't interested in doing any "crafts stuff with the ladies." Given what you know about his past leisure interests, what ideas could you suggest to Rob?

NOTES

12. How would you implement the ideas you have from Question 11?

13. What types of activity groups do you think Rob might enjoy?

Equipment/Adaptations

14. What type of adaptations would you make in Rob's room so that he could find the different clothing items in his closet and dresser (T-shirts, underwear, socks, shirts, slacks, belt, shoes)?

15. What type of adaptations would you make in the dining room to assist Rob during meals?

16. In general, what are some common environmental adaptations for people with visual impairments?

Neuromusculoskeletal

17. How would you address Rob's sensory deficits, especially as they relate to his difficulty with buttons and zippers?

18. Please describe three treatment activities that will address the sensory deficits. At least two need to be functional and purposeful activities.

Psychosocial

19. Rob gets easily frustrated and is having difficulty adjusting to his new environment. What psychosocial issues may be influencing his feelings?

20. What are Rob's strengths in this area, and how can these be incorporated into daily treatment? How can the team address these strengths together?

Patient/Family Education

21. Design a patient education program for the staff on how to work with a blind resident.

21a. What services can you find in your area for the blind? Explain how Rob might benefit from them.

Situations

22. You have given the dining room staff (both day and evening) an in-service on setting up Rob's place setting and orienting him to his meal. However, you go into the dining room to check on this and see that no one followed your in-service guidelines. You check with Rob and find out that staff is inconsistent about doing this, but that when they do what they are supposed to do, he has a much better dining experience. How do you handle this situation?

23. Similar to the situation in the dining room, you have posted signs on Rob's dresser and closet saying what clothes go where so he can find them and dress himself. You have also in-serviced the housekeeping and nursing staff. However, when checking his room, you see that his clothes are not put away as requested. How do you handle this situation?

24. Could you combine the situations in Questions 22 and 23 and address them together? What would you say, and how would you go about doing this?

NOTES

Discharge Planning

25. You are ready to discharge Rob from skilled OT, but are afraid of things slipping without regular monitoring to ensure that the techniques you have put in place are continued. Who do you think would be the best person to monitor his programs for mealtime and room organization? How would you set up this monitoring program?

NOTES

Chapter 19

Sean:
Left Above Knee Amputation,
Stage II Sacral Decubitus Ulcer

Sean is a 67-year-old Caucasian old man with a diagnosis of left above knee amputation secondary to diabetes mellitus. He also has a diagnosis of a Stage II sacral decubitus ulcer. Sean has a past medical history of alcohol abuse, depression, and status post right great toe amputation. Sean had the left leg amputated **below** the knee ten years ago. The amputation to above the knee was performed 11 weeks ago. The decubitus ulcer on his sacrum had healed from a Stage III to a Stage II while Sean was in the hospital.

Sean was transferred to the nursing home from the veteran's hospital. Sean had been living alone in the community. His daughter had come to visit from out of state and found him without food in the house, unclean, and with a sore on his buttocks and left stump. Sean thought the sore on the left leg had started when he accidentally banged his leg against the wheelchair during a transfer. His daughter thought the sore on his sacrum had probably come from poor hygiene, nutrition, and positioning. Sean had been staying in his wheelchair all day, sometimes even sleeping in it at night.

Sean has had multiple hospitalizations in the past, usually due to not caring for himself properly. Sean routinely refuses to see his doctor and will only go if his daughter drives him. "I can't understand all that garbage they tell me. That's why I need Mary to come with me. She can talk to them," he says. Sean's only daughter, Mary, is a nurse. Unfortunately, she also lives almost 2 hours away. She moved when her husband was transferred about 3 years ago. She has invited her father to come live with them, but he refuses to leave his home.

Sean has been widowed for 15 years. His wife died quickly of cancer, and he still grieves for her. Mary reports that her mother did everything for her father and upon her mother's death, her father was truly lost. Sean owns a grand home in the oldest part of the city. He says that the house has 18 rooms if you include the loft in the attic. He and his wife had planned on having a very large family but "God had other plans for us." They had only one child, Mary, to whom Sean is very close. Sean worked as a carpenter until he lost his leg 10 years ago.

Prior to his hospitalization, Sean had been able to perform his ADLs independently, but admitted he "cleans up" sporadically. Sean says he bathes and changes his clothes twice a week. He does not use the shower. He transferred independently, is nonambulatory, and moved around the house with his wheelchair. Sean is continent of bowel and bladder and uses a drop arm commode over the toilet at home. He also keeps a urinal hanging on his wheel chair to use, but will often spill the urinal while voiding or while moving around in the chair. His daughter reports throwing his wheelchair cushion away after she got him into the hospital because it was too soiled to be used again.

Sean receives Meals on Wheels from the Department of Elder Services once a day. He does not cook and relies on the microwave to heat meals, usually frozen dinners. Sean does not drive and hires a neighborhood woman to grocery shop for him. Mary says he had not called the woman for her services for almost a month before he went into the hospital. "I just don't feel that hungry anymore," he told Mary when she scolded him for not having enough food in the house.

Sean does not do housekeeping or laundry. He has a housekeeper from Elder Services in once every 2 weeks. She has offered to come more frequently, as the house needs it, but Sean refuses. Mary says the house was in the "worst shape ever" when she visited her father this last time. Sean has also let his finances go, despite his ability to manage his own money. Mary found many late notices from the gas and electric companies.

Sean is admitted to the nursing home until Mary is able to build an addition onto her home where her father can live. He has only agreed to this recently. He has insisted on going back to his own house but Mary forbids it. He agrees to move in with her only if he can have his own quarters so he will not burden her and her family.

He also will not let her use her own money to build the addition, and insists the money from the sale of his house go to cover the costs of the renovations. He wants Mary to have the rest of the money from the sale of his home as payment for his care. Mary wants him to move in right away but Sean is adamant about waiting. "I pick my battles with my father," Mary says. "He is very stubborn and if I expect to win all of them, I'm wrong!" Therefore, the plan remains for Sean to stay at the nursing home until an in-law apartment is ready for him.

While this seems like a reasonable discharge plan, the entire process is slowed by the lack of an interested buyer for Sean's house. It is large, but needs many repairs. Sean hopes it will not take too long, as he wants to "get out of institutional living!" At best, Sean and his family estimate this will be several months. Sean is to receive nursing, PT, OT, nutrition, and social services while at the facility.

Occupational Therapy Evaluation

Upon evaluation, Sean is cooperative and friendly. He seems to like to talk despite his no-nonsense attitude. He has no cognitive, perceptual, or hearing deficits. He wears bifocals for reading and distance. He has decreased sensation in the right LE and in bilateral fingertips. The amputation is still sensitive to touch, and Sean reports that sometimes even feeling his pants brush against the stump makes him quiver.

Sean has normal range and coordination in his UE. He is slightly weak in his bilateral UEs, scoring only a F+/G− overall in manual muscle testing. He says he feels like he is weaker than he was before his surgery. Sean complains of pain in his left stump only during occasional movement or touch. He reports muscle spasms in the limb and says they seem to occur at will. He describes the pain from the spasms as shooting up into the hip area. He says the ulcer pain in his sacrum is unbearable at times, and he takes pain medication for relief. Because of the location of the sore, he can only tolerate being out of bed a few hours at a time. The stump is mostly healed, and nursing is caring for the wound area. There is slight redness but no swelling.

Sean is able to roll side to side in bed and pull himself up from supine to sit with minimum assistance. He performs his transfers with contact guard to minimum assistance depending on his level of fatigue. He washes himself in bed independently except for his back, buttocks, and left stump. Although it takes him awhile, he is able to dress himself independently. Sean is not very thorough during the bathing activity. Sean can manage to cleanse the stump but has been asked by the nursing staff to allow them to do it. He states he has little interest or experience in any kitchen or homemaking tasks and refuses to partake in that portion of the evaluation. Sean spends his free time watching TV or reading.

Sean is open to having therapy but isn't sure how occupational therapy can benefit him. He states his goals are to go live with Mary and feel stronger again.

QUESTIONS

Goals/Treatment Plan

1. Write out a problem list for Sean.

2. What long-term goals would you and Sean set for his occupational therapy treatment?

3. What short-term goals would you and Sean set for his occupational therapy treatment?

4. What strengths do you feel Sean can capitalize on to help him meet his goals?

5. What obstacles do you foresee for Sean in his efforts to meet his goals?

6. Write out a specific treatment plan for Sean including frequency and duration.

Safety/Precautions

7. What precautions should be taken to prevent further skin breakdown for Sean? Write out a list and note which staff members would implement each step.

NOTES

Self-Care/Work/Leisure

8. How long do you anticipate it will be before Sean is performing his bathing independently? Why?

9. How would you address Sean's refusal to participate in the kitchen and home management portion of the evaluation?

10. How would you address Sean's lack of concern with home management and meal preparation in the past?

11. How would you assess Sean's leisure needs?

12. How, if at all, would you incorporate these needs into his treatment plan?

Equipment/Adaptations

13. What type of adaptive equipment might benefit Sean in reaching his goals?

14. Sean's daughter asks you what type of adaptations should Sean have in his apartment so she can tell the architect. What recommendations do you make?

15. Would you recommend an overhead trapeze for Sean? Why or why not?

Neuromusculoskeletal

16. Describe how you would address Sean's complaint of weakness in his UEs.

17. Give a description of a treatment session with Sean to address this issue.

18. How would you determine when Sean's strength has sufficiently improved?

19. What would you use as your benchmark point?

Psychosocial

20. What psychosocial issues do you think were affecting Sean before his hospitalization?

21. What psychosocial issues do you think are affecting Sean since his arrival at the nursing home?

22. How would you address Sean's previous lack of concern for his own care?

23. How do you think Sean's deteriorated condition has impacted Mary?

24. What impact do you think her feelings have on Sean?

25. In a skilled nursing facility, what discipline specializes in dealing with psychosocial issues?

26. Who could be used as a consultant in this case?

Patient/Family Education

27. What are topic areas in which you feel Sean needs to be educated?

28. How should the information be presented to Sean in order for him to be receptive to it?

NOTES

Situations

29. You overhear other team members laughing about how dirty the hospital said Sean was when he was admitted to the nursing home. What is your initial reaction? How do you respond and why?

30. You stop in to see Sean at lunchtime to say hello. You see he has not eaten any of his lunch. His answer is that he's not hungry. How do you respond?

31. You are assisting Sean with a transfer to the wheelchair. He complains of pain on his buttocks during the transfer. What do you do?

32. You are working on toilet transfers in the OT clinic with Sean, and he asks you to actually help him use the toilet in the bathroom. You do, and then you leave the bathroom for his privacy. After he moves his bowels, he asks to be transferred back to the chair. He tells you he already wiped himself, but since the toilet paper in out of his reach behind the sink, you doubt this is true. How do you handle this?

33. You meet Sean in his room to bring him to occupational therapy. You notice he has an odor like urine. You casually look at him to see if it looks as though his pants are wet. They don't seem to be, but you can't tell for sure. What do you do?

34. You ask Sean if he urinated in his pants and he becomes angry with you, telling you to mind your own business. How do you respond to his reaction?

35. You go to Sean's room to bring him to the therapy clinic and he has on the same clothes that he's been wearing for the last 2 days. They are stained and he has a slight odor. What might you do in this instance?

36. Sean continues to refuse to participate in any meal preparation activities, despite the fact that he'll be responsible for his own lunch preparation while Mary is at work. Since you cannot force him, what do you do?

Discharge Planning

37. Sean is discharged from OT before it is time for him to leave the facility to live with Mary. How would you ensure that Sean maintains the gains he made in OT?

38. When it comes time for Sean to leave the nursing home, what do you think should be in place to ensure a safe transition to his new home?

39. Would you recommend home OT for Sean? Why or why not?

NOTES

Chapter 20

Teresa:
End-Stage Alzheimer's Disease

Teresa is a 79-year-old Caucasian female who has been living in the skilled nursing facility for 8 years. She has a diagnosis of Alzheimer's disease, hypothyroidism, and osteoporosis. She is married, but her husband doesn't come to visit anymore, partly because of his age and partly because she doesn't recognize him and he doesn't like to see her in her current condition. He is supportive and will supply whatever the facility asks for in terms of clothing and inexpensive items (i.e., a stuffed animal). They have one daughter who lives far away, but comes to visit her parents at least four times a year and calls frequently. Currently, Teresa is in the end stages of the disease. She is nonverbal, dependent for all ADLs, is fed by a g-tube, has a foley catheter, and is non-ambulatory. She is transferred out of bed to a reclining chair daily. She used to love gardening and dogs and was very religious. She and her husband were a devoted couple. During her daughter's recent visit she was shocked at the deterioration in her mother's condition and requested that something be done to address some of the issues. Teresa was referred by her physician to occupational therapy for positioning needs and to address contractures and sensory stimulation.

Occupational Therapy Evaluation

Teresa is seen by occupational therapy while she is in bed and while she is in her recliner to address positioning needs. She opens her eyes and can make eye contact sporadically, but does not respond to any commands or questions. She moans if painful stimuli are felt. Testing for sensation and hearing were not completed. Her AROM is limited as she has contractures at the elbows, wrists, and fingers. Her shoulders may be passively ranged to 90° before she moans with pain. There is also resistance at the end of the range. Her elbows are contracted at 90° of flexion. Her wrists have contractures at 45° of flexion and her hands are fisted. The contractures can all be passively stretched an additional 10°–15°, but no more. The contractures in her UE make it difficult for staff to bathe Teresa. Her hands have a foul odor because they have not been properly cleansed. Teresa also has LE contractures, hips 100° flexion, knees contracted at 45°, and plantar flexion contracture at 35°. Her knees can be passively ranged to −10° extension. She has increased tone in the hip adductors, which make it difficult to separate her legs for cleansing and catheter care. Teresa's positioning in the recliner is difficult. She is propped up by pillows on all sides and still slips down in the recliner. She has to be reclined all the way, but this puts her neck into hyperextension. She also leans more to the left side. Currently, it takes two nursing assistants to wash and dress Teresa due to the tightness of her limbs. She is transferred by a Hoyer lift. The goal for OT is to properly position Teresa both in and out of bed, address the PROM and contractures so that daily care can be more easily given, and provide sensory stimulation.

QUESTIONS

Goals/Treatment Plan

1. What would your long- and short-term goals be for Teresa?

2. Write out a problem list for Teresa.

3. What frame of reference would you use for each of your goals?

4. What aspects of the treatment can be done by a COTA? By a rehab aide? By an OT aide?

Safety/Precautions

5. What precautions do you have to take when doing PROM with Teresa? Why?

6. What is a Hoyer lift, and how do you use one?

Self-Care/Work/Leisure

7. How might you incorporate some of Teresa's past leisure interests into your treatment sessions?

8. Because Teresa is dependent in her self-care, what is the role of OT in this area?

9. Because Teresa is unable to ambulate, what are the problems that are associated with prolonged immobility? How would you address some of these in OT treatment?

10. How is skin breakdown prevented in a patient in Teresa's dependent condition?

11. How do you address the foul smell of Teresa's hands? What do you think causes this smell?

Equipment/Adaptations

12. What types of adaptations might you suggest to properly position Teresa while she is in bed?

13. What is the optimal seating positioning for Teresa when she is out of bed?

14. What do you see as the major obstacles to properly positioning Teresa when she is out of bed? Would you suggest any different types of seating systems? Remember, insurance rarely allows for specialized wheelchairs for nursing-home residents.

15. Look at a catalogue and see if there is any positioning equipment that might help to position Teresa properly when she is out of bed. What is the cost of this equipment? Who do you think would pay for it? Do you think the amount of money you are asking for is reasonable for the benefits it may have?

Neuromusculoskeletal

16. Teresa has many contractures. How would you address each one of her contractures in a comprehensive program?

17. If you chose to use splints, what type of splint would you make initially and why? What material would you make this splint out of?

18. What would be the wearing schedule for the splints?

NOTES

19. Look at a catalogue of splints. What kind could you purchase instead of make? What would be the advantage of purchasing a splinting device over making one? Why did you choose the splint(s) that you did?

20. Describe optimal bed positions for Teresa in supine and side-lying.

21. What are the major obstacles to positioning Teresa properly when she is in bed?

22. What would the benefits of PROM be for Teresa?

23. How often would you recommend that Teresa receive PROM each day? Who will be responsible for doing this?

24. Describe a sensory stimulation program for Teresa. Who would carry out this program and how often should it be done?

Patient/Family Education

25. What would be important to educate staff about in relation to Teresa's occupational therapy plan of care?

26. How would you go about this education process?

Situations

27. You go in to check on Teresa's splints and find that they are on totally wrong. You have put a sign on the wall by her bed telling the staff how to apply the splints, but they are not done correctly. You check with the nursing assistant assigned to Teresa and discover that English is not her primary language. What do you do?

28. During PROM with Teresa, you feel a slight "click" during shoulder ROM. You notice that Teresa starts to moan as if she is in pain during this ranging activity, and she never did before. What do you think might have happened and why? What do you do?

29. One day, you notice that Teresa does not have one of the positioning devices on her chair. What do you do?

Discharge Planning

30. You are about to discharge Teresa from skilled OT services. Does Medicare allow you to monitor her on a regular basis? If so, how often will you put in your discharge plan that you want to do this? If not, how will you ensure that all your splints and positioning devices are used and used correctly?

NOTES

Part VI

Outpatient Rehabilitation Clinic

Chapter 21

Ursula:
Right Carpal Tunnel Repair,
Left Carpal Tunnel Syndrome

Ursula is a 44-year-old African-American female with a diagnosis of carpal tunnel syndrome. She works as a hairdresser in a busy salon in an urban area. By her lunch break Ursula had been noticing a tingling in her right hand that usually went away by the time lunch was over. After a few weeks, she became aware that, by evening, her right hand was tingling and felt like it had "fallen asleep". She started to drop silverware when trying to prepare dinner. By bedtime, her right arm would be feeling tired and painful. At first, the symptoms disappeared by morning, but soon she noticed that her right hand and arm hurt all the time, some times more than others. On a few occasions, she almost dropped the hair dryer out of her hand when she was drying a client's hair. After this happened a few times, she decided to see her primary care physician, who suggested she wear a wrist support that she could buy at the local pharmacy. This helped for a short time, but the symptoms never completely went away. Ursula was then referred to a hand specialist who tried anti-inflammatory medications, a custom-made splint, and rest for a week. This also helped, but as soon as she returned to work, the symptoms returned. Ursula did not wear the splint at work because it hindered her use of the scissors and hair dryer. The hand specialist recommended surgery to release the nerve compression and alleviate the symptoms. In the meantime, Ursula also had symptoms of carpal tunnel syndrome in her left hand, but the physician felt that since this was in the early stages, it could be treated more conservatively.

Ursula is a married mother of four children. Her husband works as a factory foreman. Her children are between the ages of 8 and 16. She rents her chair from the salon owner and needs to show a certain number of clients in order to make it worth the rent she pays for the chair. This requires that she work 6 days a week. She takes only a lunch break and a short cigarette break in the morning and afternoon each day. Ursula can make her own hours, but she has to let the receptionist know what hours she will be working each week.

Her husband and she share the responsibilities of the household, and the two older children contribute by doing laundry and cleaning the house. Ursula and her husband share the cooking, grocery shopping, and duties of getting the children wherever they have to go. Although their schedules don't allow a lot of time together, Ursula and her husband are very close and make sure that Sunday is a family day.

Ursula is a deeply religious woman. She enjoys her work as a hairdresser and she is also an active church volunteer. Her children all are active in the church youth group as well. Ursula and her husband enjoy bowling and in the winter try to bowl one night a week.

Ursula is an energetic woman with an upbeat disposition and outlook on life. She came from a large southern family and was one of the youngest, so there is not much that bothers her. She states she gets her strength from her church and family.

She was referred to outpatient occupational therapy 2 weeks after the surgery for her right hand and to address the deteriorating function of the left hand. Ursula's goals are to return to work at her previous level in 2 weeks. She says that if she doesn't pay the rent on the chair, the salon owner will just rent it out to someone else. There are a lot of hairdressers who want to be in this salon.

Occupational Therapy Evaluation

Ursula has no deficits in cognition, perception, hearing, or vision. She has sensory deficits for light touch, deep pressure, hot/cold, and sharp/dull along the median nerve distribution of both hands, with the right hand being worse than the left. Ursula is right-handed. Formal testing using the Moberg Pickup Test and the Jebsen Hand Function Test showed a significant decrease in fine-motor coordination. Strength was tested on the left hand with a dynamometer and registered 25 pounds. The right hand was not tested due to the recent surgery. Her AROM in both UEs is WFL. However, the strength in her right shoulder is 3+/5. Her left shoulder is 4/5; both elbows are 4/5. Ursula reports some pain at the right wrist where the surgery was performed, but it occurs mostly with activity. Her left wrist and hand continue to have paresthesia upon wrist flexion. Both hands have decreased pinch strength for two point, three point, and lateral pinches. Ursula has slight edema of the right hand and fingers.

Ursula is independent in functional mobility and all transfers. She has difficulty with ADLs, especially tasks that require fine-motor skills. Ursula's husband or daughters have been helping her get dressed since the surgery. She needs help with her bra, tying shoes, buttons, zippers, and socks. She has difficulty washing but will not let anyone help her. Meal preparation is difficult and her husband and children have been doing it since her surgery. Housework is also being done by her family, and Ursula feels bad about her inability to do it herself.

She is very anxious to get better and says she will comply with any program that she is given. Her family is very supportive. Ursula's goals are to get back to the salon in 2 weeks; to be able to dress, shower, and cleanse herself; and to be pain free and able to care for her family and her home.

QUESTIONS

Goals/Treatment Plan

1. What are your long- and short-term goals for Ursula?

2. What is the first priority to address in Ursula's treatment and why?

3. What aspects of Ursula's treatment program could a COTA be responsible for?

4. What, if any, obstacles do you see to Ursula's recovery? How might you address these?

5. What strengths does Ursula bring to her treatment sessions?

Safety/Precautions

6. What are some precautions to take when working with Ursula?

Self-Care/Work/Leisure

7. How will you address Ursula's dressing deficits while working in an outpatient department?

8. Do an activity analysis of Ursula's job as a hairdresser.

9. What level of hand function does Ursula need to return to her job?

10. What home management tasks will be difficult for Ursula to do for the next month?

11. What home management tasks will Ursula be able to do within 2 weeks, and will these tasks need modifications? If so, what will these modifications be?

12. Ursula talked about her leisure interests during the initial evaluation. What are they, and how will her carpal tunnel syndrome affect her ability to pursue them?

NOTES

Equipment/Adaptations

13. What, if any, adaptive equipment would Ursula benefit from for self-care tasks? What is the cost of this equipment?

14. What, if any, adaptive equipment would Ursula benefit from for meal preparation? What is the cost of this equipment?

15. Ursula's carpal tunnel syndrome occurred due to her job. What, if any, modifications or adaptations would you suggest she adopt at work? Why?

16. Can you find ergonomic tools in a catalogue or store for Ursula to start using? What is their cost? If you can't find any, how might you adapt those tools she already has to prevent further cumulative trauma disorder?

17. What adaptations would you suggest Ursula make in her daily routine as it applies to her job?

Neuromusculoskeletal

18. Carpal tunnel syndrome involves which nerve, and what are the motor and sensory distributions of this nerve?

19. Please write out a protocol for Ursula to follow to control the edema in her fingers.

20. Please write out a home exercise program for Ursula to follow for weeks 1 and 2 of outpatient therapy. What type of exercises will you prescribe and why?

21. Ursula has the beginnings of carpal tunnel syndrome in her left hand, and her doctor wishes to treat it without surgery. What treatment will you use for her left hand?

22. What is the purpose of wearing a splint for carpal tunnel syndrome?

23. What type of splint, if any, will you make for Ursula, and what material will you use? Please write out a wearing schedule for the splint for week 1. How will this differ from week 2 and beyond?

24. Ursula has some significant sensory deficits in her right hand. How will you address these in your treatment sessions? Will you suggest any home activities for her, and, if so, what will they be?

25. While doing some gross-motor coordination activities, you notice that Ursula is able to reach the object, but she is moving her whole body, her shoulder is elevated, and abducted when she goes to reach. What is the most likely cause of this and what will you do to address this?

26. What type of purposeful activities can you use to address Ursula's fine-motor deficits?

27. What is the role of physical agent modalities in occupational therapy? Can COTAs use them? Who is responsible for establishing competency for the use of these modalities?

28. What, if any, physical agent modalities would you use during Ursula's treatment program? Why would you use these modalities, and how would you address their use in relation to purposeful activity?

Psychosocial

29. Ursula is having a difficult time coping with her recovery. She feels it is going too slowly and that the doctor lied to her about how fast it would take her to recover. She is getting discouraged and saying things like "I'll have to give up my chair at the salon." She has also noted that she is doing her home exercise program when she feels like it, "since it doesn't seem to be helping any." How will you address her psychological state?

NOTES

Patient/Family Education

30. Ursula doesn't understand what carpal tunnel syndrome is or why she has it. Create a patient information booklet for her and her family.

31. What types of hand and wrist movements should be avoided for someone who has carpal tunnel syndrome?

Situations

32. Ursula usually comes to therapy alone, but one day her husband accompanies her to see how her therapy is going. It is a typical busy day and you are seeing two patients at a time. While one is doing an activity, you are working with the other. The patients are close enough so that you can monitor them at the same time. This is not unusual at your clinic. At the end of the treatment session, Ursula's husband pulls you aside and angrily accuses you of spending more time with the other patient you were seeing than with Ursula and says you did that because the other patient is "richer" than Ursula. How do you handle this situation?

Discharge Planning

33. Ursula is to be discharged from outpatient therapy after 4 weeks. She has made gains in all areas of ROM, strength grasp, and pinch strength, but these have not returned to what they should be for her age and profession. Her sensory deficits, although still present, do not bother her that much. She can dress herself, but her hands are still fatigued by the end of the day. What type of home program will you send home with Ursula, and how will you impress on her the importance of her following it?

34. Write a discharge note to Ursula's hand surgeon.

NOTES

Chapter 22

Violet:
Right Flexor Tendon Laceration,
Depression

Violet is a 31-year-old Caucasian female with a diagnosis of a right wrist flexor tendon laceration following a suicide attempt. Violet also has a diagnosis of depression. She had never attempted suicide before. Violet, or Vi as she prefers to be called, is referred to outpatient occupational therapy by her hand surgeon.

Vi had become distraught after her parents threatened to "disown" her if she went ahead with her plans to marry a man outside of her faith. Vi's family is Roman Catholic and her fiancé is Jewish. Initially her boyfriend Keith said he was willing to convert to Catholicism, but decided against it when he met with resistance from his parents. Keith told Violet that they would not be able to get married unless she converted to Judaism. Vi felt as though she could not bear the loss of her boyfriend, her parents, or her religion and slit her right wrist with a kitchen knife. Her mother found her and called 911; Vi was brought into the emergency room. She was operated on by a hand surgeon with the goal of full use of her right hand. Vi was then hospitalized for a week and a half on the med-pysch unit of the hospital.

Vi works as a bookkeeper for her father's furniture business. She has worked at this position since she graduated from high school. Vi did not go to college because it would have meant leaving her position at the store. Every mention of leaving results in her father either begging her not to leave or threatening to cut her off financially. Vi lives with her parents and has no siblings.

Vi dated rarely, and Keith is her first real romantic relationship. He had worked at her father's store until the two started dating; he decided to quit to avoid the comments from Violet's father. The two tentatively plan to marry in 6 months. Both sets of parents object strongly to the union.

During her psychiatric stay, Violet was given a dorsal blocking splint, which she wore 24 hours a day. On orders from the physician, the charge nurse instructed the mental health workers to assist Vi in following a post-surgery Duran protocol that was to be carried out every hour. The protocol included passive finger flexion (MCP, PIP, DIP, and composition) and active extension into the splint to protect the repair and promote movement. Vi exercised only if she was reminded to do so.

Vi had no functional limitations prior to the suicide attempt. Since her discharge from the inpatient facility, Violet is scheduled to see a psychiatrist three times per week on an outpatient basis. This is her first time in counseling and first time on antidepressants. She had her sutures removed 2 weeks after the surgery. When she came to the outpatient department, it had been 2½ weeks since the attempt and resultant injury. She is scheduled to see the hand surgeon again in 3 days.

Occupational Therapy Evaluation

Upon evaluation, Violet exhibits no hearing, visual, sensory, or perceptual limitations. She responds to questions slowly, as if she has limited energy to answer. Her voice is soft and frail. Vi has no long-term memory deficits, but does display some difficulty with immediate recall and short-term memory. This appears to be due to a decreased attention span and inability to focus on the conversation.

Violet is left-handed. She has no physical limitations other than those related to the tendon laceration. Violet has active right digit extension as follows: 50° MCP, −20° PIP, and full DIP extension. Passively, she has

60° MCP flexion and 40° PIP flexion contractures beginning with the ability to move only half range to distal palmer crease. She has 30° DIP flexion passively. Vi has slight edema in all digits and the skin appears fragile and glossy. Violet denies pain or discomfort while wearing the splint. She reports doing her exercises faithfully, but it is apparent this is not so.

Vi is independent in mobility. She reports independence in self-care and says the OT at the hospital taught her how to get dressed and wash with one hand. Vi says she has been doing almost everything that she had been before except cooking (due to lack of appetite), cleaning (due to disinterest), and working. Vi also reports not driving at this time. She states she simply avoids two-handed tasks and does things slowly with her left hand.

Vi wants to regain full use of her right hand so she "won't look like a freak." Vi says, unenthusiastically, that she will participate in OT as her doctor ordered. Her affect remains sad throughout the evaluation. Her next appointment for occupational therapy is set for the day after Violet's visit to the doctor.

QUESTIONS

Goals/Treatment Plan

1. What questions would you have for the hand surgeon before designing Violet's OT treatment plan?

2. How would you get these answers from the physician?

3. Write out a problem list for Violet.

4. What are Violet's strengths, and how could those be tapped into in order to further her treatment?

5. What long-term goals would you and Violet set for occupational therapy treatment?

6. What short-term goals would you and Violet set for occupational therapy treatment?

7. If the hand surgeon orders active wrist flexion within the splint in addition to the present protocol, how would this change your treatment plan?

Safety/Precautions

8. What specific precautions should Violet follow to protect her tendon repair?

9. What could happen if she does not follow these precautions?

10. What other issues might develop if Violet does not follow her exercise protocols?

11. How could you reinforce Violet's adherence to precautions?

Self-Care/Work/Leisure

12. How would you address the absence of Violet's work role?

13. Violet tells you her father wants her to come back to work right away. She asks if you could explain her situation to him so he won't force her back too soon. What do you say to her in response?

14. Do you think Violet is physically and/or emotionally ready to return to her job at this time? Explain why or why not.

NOTES

Equipment/Adaptations

15. If Violet was to return to work now, what type of accommodations would need to be made for her?

16. Explain to Violet how to care for her dorsal blocking splint.

Neuromusculoskeletal

17. At this point, would you be working on strengthening with Violet? Why or why not?

18. Write out a home exercise program for Violet.

19. Explain your treatment techniques related to scar management.

20. Explain your treatment techniques related to edema management.

21. Be prepared to describe to the class with a demonstration how the ROM exercises would be carried out.

Cognition/Perception

22. How might you incorporate treatment of Violet's decreased attention span and recall into your hand therapy sessions?

Psychosocial

23. How might this injury have affected Violet's relationship with her parents?

24. What impact will the relationship with her parents have on Violet's progress?

25. How might this injury have affected Violet's relationship with her fiancé? What impact will that have on her progress?

26. Do you feel it is appropriate to address Violet's depression in outpatient OT? Why or why not?

Patient/Family Education

27. Violet's father accompanies her to one of her OT sessions. He stands up and demands that you explain to him why his daughter is not "allowed" to return to work. What do you do?

28. Violet's father starts blaming you for her slow progress. His voice is escalating, and Violet starts to cry. What do you do?

29. How could you prevent this from happening again?

30. How would you educate Violet's family about her injury and recovery process?

Situations

31. Violet's doctor now tells her that she is allowed active digit flexion within the splint. How will this change your treatment plan and goals?

32. Violet is minimally compliant with her exercises and home program. Why might this be?

33. How could you help improve her follow-through with her home program?

NOTES

34. Violet has cancelled the last two OT sessions. What do you do?

35. Violet's PIP contractures improve very little. What would your course of action be?

36. What might the hand surgeon decide to do at that point?

37. How might his decision affect Violet's psychological status? Her physical status?

Discharge Planning

38. Violet's progress is at a plateau. However, when you begin to speak of discharge, she promises to work harder. Explain your reaction toward her promise. Describe what you would say to her, and what your next course of action would be?

39. What would your feelings be regarding Violet's discharge from therapy?

NOTES

Chapter 23

Walter:
Right 2–5 Digit Amputation

Walter is a 32-year-old Caucasian man with a diagnosis of amputations of the right 2–5 digits. The amputation occurred in the 2nd and 3rd digits at the PIP joints. The 4th digit was severed at the distal end of the proximal phalanx. His 5th digit was amputated just above the MCP joint. Walter had no other medical problems or conditions before this accident. The accident occurred at home; he had been building a deck for the back of his house. He had borrowed his brother's table saw and was working in his cellar. Walter can't recall exactly how it happened, but the accident resulted in the loss of 4 digits.

Walter had no limitations prior to his accident. He works full time as a social worker for the Department of Youth Services, working with troubled adolescents. He is gifted in his work and has helped many teens turn themselves around. Walter also attends graduate school in the evenings, studying to be a psychologist. He lives with Stuart, his significant other. He plays softball weekly and is the co-captain of his team. He and Stuart live in a rural area in a small two-bedroom home.

His hand surgeon referred Walter to outpatient therapy. It has been almost 2½ weeks since the accident. Walter is eager to get started with therapy and hopeful regarding the outcome. Walter has a follow-up appointment with the hand surgeon next week. His goals for therapy are to use his hand "as though nothing ever happened."

Occupational Therapy Evaluation

Upon evaluation, Walter exhibits no cognitive, perceptual, visual, or hearing deficits. Walter reports experiencing intermittent sensations of his fingers being fully attached. He reports this is stronger and more prevalent on the ulnar side of his hand. He has hypersensitivity on the tips where the amputations occurred. Walter wears a sterile dressing over the entire hand and removes it for the evaluation. Walter is right-hand dominant.

Walter has marked edema and redness throughout the hand, more predominantly in the palmar region. The edema limits his thumb ROM, especially in opposition. He is unable to oppose his digits and can only touch the 2nd digit on the lateral side in a lateral pinch. He has approximately 5°–8° flexion at the 2nd–4th MCP joints. No extension is present and abduction is minimal.

Walter has eschar formations on the 4th and 5th digits. He has healing areas on the 2nd and 3rd digits, but the skin is red and fragile and the head of the phalanx proximal is protruding from the tip of the 2nd digit. Walter reports it feeling like his skin is going to tear when he moves the 2nd finger. Walter grimaces in pain and disgust several times during the evaluation.

Walter has no other physical limitations because of the accident. He ambulates independently and reports independence with all self-care tasks, albeit with difficulty and tediousness. "I'm wearing sweatpants and sweatshirts to make it easy on myself," he states. Walter also wears slip-on sandals for easy dressing. He reports difficulty feeding himself, since he is not left-handed. Stuart assists him by cutting his food. While he appreciates it, he hates to ask him for help. They had shared in the cooking and housekeeping tasks, but Stuart has taken over all tasks. Walter is particularly concerned about his inability to write. He agrees to do "whatever is necessary" to use his hand again. He is motivated for therapy and eager to begin.

QUESTIONS

Goals/Treatment Plan

1. Devise a problem list for Walter.

2. What are Walter's strengths?

3. What specific long- and short-term goals would you set with Walter for his occupational therapy treatment?

4. How could Walter utilize his strengths to meet his goals?

5. Write out a specific treatment plan for Walter including frequency and duration.

Safety/Precautions

6. What precautions must you use when working with Walter given his condition?

7. How would these precautions be different for Walter as compared to any other patient?

8. What are some safety concerns you might have to be aware of when doing treatment with Walter?

Self-Care/Work/Leisure

9. What recommendation might you make to Walter so that he can perform bathing and dressing easier than he has been?

10. Walter tells you he'll need to wear dress shirts and pants once he returns to work. What tips can you give him to make that easier for him as well?

11. Walter states Stuart has offered to do all the cooking and housekeeping from now on. He says he is afraid Stuart will resent him for it in the future. What is your response?

12. Walter's leisure activity is softball. How will this accident affect his leisure roles? How could he still participate in this activity?

13. How will this accident affect Walter's vocational role?

14. How will this accident affect Walter's role as a student?

15. What could be done in each of these instances to return Walter to his previous level of ability in his various roles?

Equipment/Adaptations

16. What type of adaptive equipment will Walter need in order to resume self-care, work, and leisure roles? How much will this equipment cost?

Neuromusculoskeletal

17. Write out a protocol to treat Walter's sensory problems.

18. Write out a plan to address Walter's edematous hand.

19. Write out an exercise plan for Walter's occupational therapy treatment session. Be sure to include types of exercises and rationale for each.

NOTES

20. Write out a home exercise plan for Walter including the frequency in which he should perform exercises. What role would Physical Agent Modalities play in Walter's treatment? Who is qualified to administer them?

Psychosocial

21. What do you suppose the psychological impact of the amputations has been on Walter?

22. What impact do you think this will have on Stuart? Why?

Patient/Family Education

23. What are ongoing educational needs that Walter has regarding the amputations?

24. Explain how you will teach Walter how to care for his amputations.

25. Explain how you will educate yourself regarding proper care of the dressing following every OT visit.

26. How involved do you think his partner should be in the rehabilitation process? Why?

Situations

27. Walter comes in for therapy and you remove the dressing. He has obviously been bleeding a little bit from the tip of the 2nd digit. What do you do?

28. Walter tells you the phantom pain continues to distract him during the day. He describes it as burning pain in the parts of the fingers that aren't there. What type of treatment might be helpful in this instance?

29. Walter has developed a painful neuroma on the ulnar side of his hand, over the 5th MCP joint. What treatment techniques might be suggested to deal with the neuroma?

30. Walter has less edema and can now oppose his 2nd and 3rd digits on the anterior side. He wants to start practicing writing. What goals must he first meet before he can begin this type of treatment?

31. You are doing some massage of Walter's hand. Some of the eschar begins to come loose. What do you do?

32. Walter has progressed to 45° flexion in the MCPs of the 2nd and 3rd digits. He has made little gains in extension, however. How can you explain this?

33. Walter tells you he wants to start driving again. He has a standard car. What can occupational therapy do to help Walter meet his goal of driving again?

Discharge Planning

34. When will you know it is time to discharge Walter from therapy? Be specific.

35. Write out an OT program for Walter to follow after discharge from outpatient therapy.

36. Write a discharge note to send to Walter's physician.

NOTES

Chapter 24

Xavier:
Bilateral Tendonitis

Xavier is a 33-year-old man of Hispanic descent. He has a diagnosis of bilateral tendonitis, or more specifically, lateral epicondylitis. He has no other significant medical history or problems. His primary physician referred him for outpatient occupational therapy. Xavier reportedly has been experiencing worsening pain over the last 4 months. He works as a printer for a large commercial printing company. He is married with twin boys, age 8, and his wife is expecting their third child. Xavier is obviously angry about the onset of the tendonitis. He is not blaming anyone for it, but is clearly disgusted that he has pain that is slowing him down. Xavier prides himself on being a good worker.

Xavier is experiencing no functional limitations at home as a result of the tendonitis, but is worried about how much longer he is going to be able to perform at his current job. Xavier has given up his favorite activity, working out at the gym, because of his elbow pain. He says he uses ice on his elbows at night, which seems to help "a bit."

Xavier has been a printer for 13 years. He had taken a new job running a large press almost a year ago. He says that when he first began, he noticed the discomfort in his elbows. "I thought I just had to get stronger to be able to deal with lifting the paper," he says. Still, after a year of working, frequent trips to the gym, and taking vitamins, Xavier reports the pain to be increasingly worse.

Xavier operates a 40-inch press. He states that loading the paper into the press causes him the most pain. Xavier describes having to lift 40-inch wide paper off skids from the floor onto a platform on the press. He lifts the paper in increments of approximately 30 pounds at a time, up to 3,000 to 4,000 pounds a day. He also has to "fan" the paper out to allow air in between the sheets before it is printed on. Xavier explains this step as essential because without it, the paper will stick together and the press will jam. The motion of "fanning" the paper starts in pronation and moves through supination to the end range.

Xavier says he first started with pain much worse in the right arm; now his left arm feels just as bad, and the pain sometimes wakes him up at night. He says that sometimes after a particularly busy workday he will be awakened at night from the pain. Xavier remarks that it is inconsistent, however, and occasionally wakes him up at night during the weekends as well.

Xavier is responsible for all home repair, car maintenance, and yard work at home. He and his family live in a large house in the suburbs. His wife is a stay at home mom, who is responsible for all the housekeeping and child care. Xavier reports pain at times when playing ball with his sons.

Occupational Therapy Evaluation

Xavier is seen for an occupational therapy evaluation. He has no cognitive, perceptual, visual, hearing, or sensory deficits. He has AROM in normal ranges for bilateral UEs, although he reports pain during wrist extension and supination. Despite the pain, his strength is also normal. Xavier is right-handed and has no coordination deficits, edema, or skin changes.

Xavier is independent in all self-care and work tasks. He has lost no time from his work because of the tendonitis, although he reports wanting to leave early many days because of the pain. He continues driving and had not experienced inability in doing any of his normal daily tasks. Xavier's goal from therapy is to be pain-free. He agrees to participate in occupational therapy and apologized for his "crankiness." Xavier remarks, "I'm tired of dealing with this pain."

QUESTIONS

Goals/Treatment Plan

1. Write a problem list for Xavier.

2. What are Xavier's strengths?

3. What would you and Xavier set for his short-term goals? His long-term goals?

4. How could Xavier's strengths be used to help him achieve his goals?

5. Write out a treatment plan for Xavier including frequency and duration.

6. Xavier's insurance wants justification for the services you are requesting. Write out a paragraph to explain what you plan to do, why it is necessary, and what you expect to accomplish over the next 2 weeks.

Safety/Precautions

7. What precautions should Xavier take to lessen his pain?

8. What precautions should Xavier take to prevent furthering his tendonitis?

Self-Care/Work/Leisure

9. Aside from leaving his job, what might be done to make his work less likely to exacerbate the tendonitis?

10. Xavier would like to continue his workouts at the gym 3 days per week. What do you suggest?

Equipment/Adaptations

11. How might Xavier's work station and work demands be adapted to allow the healing of his tendonitis?

Neuromusculoskeletal

12. What types of Physical Agents Modalities would you use to treat Xavier's tendonitis? Explain why and who is qualified to administer them.

13. Explain the type of treatment program you would recommend for Xavier during his outpatient visits. Be specific.

14. Write out a home program for Xavier to follow. Be sure to include all information needed for a thorough, effective home program.

Psychosocial

15. Why do you think Xavier is angry about having tendonitis?

16. What other feelings might Xavier have in relation to the tendonitis?

17. Why is it so important psychologically for Xavier to have this treatment be successful?

18. What impact would it have on Xavier if his tendonitis continued?

NOTES

Patient/Family Education

19. What important things must you educate Xavier on for better treatment success?

20. Why is it important to educate Xavier regarding his part in the treatment program?

Situations

21. Xavier is making good progress and reporting less pain following 1 week of treatment. His insurance company wants to limit him to only one more visit. Explain what you would do.

22. The insurance company case manager tells you she thought Xavier was going to be having PT and not OT and wants him to change to physical therapy. What do you say and do?

23. You ask Xavier if he is following his home program and he answers, "As much as I can, but it doesn't seem like enough." What do you say?

24. Xavier asks you how much longer he has to continue with his home program. What is your response?

25. Xavier tells you he has been trying to keep his tendonitis a secret from his employers. He asks you if you think this is a good idea. What is your response? Why?

Discharge Planning

26. How long would you anticipate seeing Xavier for OT treatment if he continues with his current job?

27. If Xavier reported his pain to be present, but less pronounced, what would you recommend for him to do to meet his goals of being pain-free?

NOTES

Chapter 25

Yolanda:
Left Fractured Humerus,
2 Weeks Post-Injury

Yolanda is a 62-year-old Caucasian female who fell and sustained a proximal oblique fracture of the shaft of her left humerus while out birdwatching. Additional diagnoses include diverticulitis, osteoporosis, and ETOH abuse. Yolanda is an avid birdwatcher and goes out with friends several mornings a week to different areas. She was walking along a wooded path looking through her binoculars when she tripped and fell over a log. She put out her left arm to stop the fall (the right was holding the binoculars) and heard a crack as soon as she landed. The pain was excruciating, and her friends immediately took her to the nearest emergency room. X-rays showed a fracture of the upper humerus. Her arm was placed in a sling and no surgery was required, but the fracture is too high to immobilize with a cast.

Prior to her accident, Yolanda had no deficits in her daily life. She drove, cooked, shopped, and took care of the family finances. She has been married to her second husband for 15 years and has two grown children from her first marriage. She and her husband, Bob, enjoy traveling and entertaining. She lives in a large two-story suburban home and does not work. Her husband is an investment banker and they are well-off financially. Yolanda's children both live nearby, but are working mothers with teenaged children of their own. Although they are close, she feels her children need to live their own lives.

Yolanda has a history of alcohol abuse, but claims she has stopped drinking. She is a personable woman, but is very private and does not like to talk about herself or her family. She has always felt that she is an independent woman, who enjoys the company of others, especially women, but does not want to rely on anyone except her husband.

Yolanda is 2 weeks post-fracture and will be seen in the outpatient clinic for OT to address the fractured humerus, with discharge to her own care when therapy is complete.

Occupational Therapy Evaluation

Yolanda has no perceptual, visual, or hearing deficits, although she wears glasses for reading. Sensation is intact, although she complains of occasional tingling in her hand. She appears somewhat forgetful during the evaluation, and it is difficult to get a good history of events from her.

Yolanda is right-handed and expresses relief that it is her left arm that is broken, not the right. Strength cannot be assessed due to nonweight-bearing precautions. There is a bruise on left her upper arm and some bruises on her knees and shins from her fall. Her skin is otherwise intact. Yolanda has pain with movement of the shoulder in flexion beyond 25° and extension beyond 10°. Her arm is immobilized in a sling except for showering, dressing, and therapy for at least 2 more weeks. She has AROM in her elbow 0–110° before pain, wrist and fingers are WNL. Coordination is impaired due to immobilization. Her right arm shows no deficits in strength, ROM, or coordination.

Yolanda has difficulty getting up from low furniture, but has found that if she sits in a chair with arms she can get up more easily. She has difficulty in general with going from sit to stand or supine to stand because of her inability to use her left arm to assist. She requires assistance with dressing and fasteners. She has figured out how to brush her teeth and comb her hair, but can't put it in a bun, like she normally wears it. She has permission to shower, but has been to fearful to try it. She is dependent for all meal preparation, but reports that she has a housekeeper who does that if she needs her to, or else she and her husband go out to eat.

Yolanda considers her fracture to be a stupid accident and a great inconvenience. She and her husband have a 4-week trip coming up in 3 weeks and she doesn't want to be hampered with a sling and pain. She gives her goals as returning to her previous activity level and of being recovered enough to at least go away without the sling. Her doctor's orders are for pendulum exercises for 1 week progressing to active-assistive and active exercises as tolerated.

QUESTIONS

Goals/Treatment Plan

1. What are your long- and short-term goals for Yolanda? Write out a treatment plan for Yolanda based on a 3-week timetable.

2. What obstacles do you see in working with Yolanda?

3. What strengths does she bring to therapy?

4. What frame of reference will you use in treatment and why?

Safety/Precautions

5. What precautions must you take in working with Yolanda and why?

6. Yolanda has a history of alcohol abuse. Is this important to know and, if so, why?

7. Are there any safety concerns regarding Yolanda's ability to function at home?

Self-Care/Work/Leisure

8. What are Yolanda's self-care deficits, and how will you address these in an outpatient setting?

9. Yolanda has told you that she hasn't taken a shower yet because she is afraid of the pain when her arm is out of the sling. How can you work with her on this so the outcome is that she takes a shower at home?

10. Yolanda usually wears her hair in a bun or pulled back off her face. Her hair length is past her shoulders. She is very frustrated that she cannot wear it as she usually does; it makes her feel unkempt. How can you address this issue?

Equipment/Adaptations

11. What types of difficulties do you anticipate Yolanda might have at mealtime? What adaptive equipment would you recommend, and how much would it cost?

12. What types of difficulties do you anticipate Yolanda might have with dressing and showering? What adaptive equipment would you recommend, and how much would it cost?

Neuromusculoskeletal

13. According to the physician's initial orders, what types of exercises will you do with Yolanda during the first week? What are these, and why do you do them?

14. When would you test the AROM of Yolanda's left UE?

NOTES

15. Would you give Yolanda activities/exercises for her left hand? Why or why not?

16. Her physician ordered AAROM and AROM activities starting at week 2. Write out a home exercise program for Yolanda that follows these orders.

17. What type of treatment activities would you start doing in week 2? Please choose four and explain why you would do these.

Psychosocial

18. At 3 weeks post-fracture, Yolanda becomes very teary during her treatment sessions, but will not open up to tell you why. How do you handle this?

19. Yolanda tells you that she continues to take the pain medication (Percocet) three times a day because she is afraid of having pain. Should this concern you? If so, why and what do you do about it?

Patient/Family Education

20. Yolanda has a diagnosis that may have contributed to her fracture. What is it, and what should she know about its relationship to her humeral fracture?

21. What patient education does Yolanda need in relation to her fracture?

Situations

22. Yolanda spends a lot of her leisure time socializing and feels the sling she has been given looks ugly; she has decided not to wear it. She says that she can hold her arm still. How do you address this issue?

23. By the third week of treatment, Yolanda has missed her first two appointments. When you call her to see why, she says that she is doing the exercises and that she has more to do to get ready for her trip in 1 week. How do you handle this? Is it important for her to come in for the next two appointments? Why or why not?

Discharge Planning

24. Yolanda is ready to be discharged. Her arm has just come out of the sling, and she and her husband are leaving on their trip next week. She is still very weak in her left shoulder and her gross-motor coordination is mildly impaired due to the shoulder weakness. What type of program do you give her upon discharge, and what are your discharge instructions to her?

NOTES

Part VII

Home and Community Healthcare

Chapter 26

Zoe:
Rheumatoid Arthritis,
Obsessive-Compulsive Disorder

Zoe is a 68-year-old Caucasian woman with a diagnosis of rheumatoid arthritis (RA), insulin-dependent diabetes, and obsessive-compulsive disorder (OCD). She has had RA since she was 45 years old, with a history of exacerbations and remissions with progressively worsening deformities of her hands, her left hand being worse than her right. Zoe is divorced, has no children, and no contact with her former husband. Her OCD has been under control with medication; however, she still fusses over her environment. She worked as an administrative assistant in a doctor's office for 25 years until her arthritis made it difficult for her to continue working and she retired a year and a half ago.

Zoe lives alone with her cats, Maple and Poppy. She lives on the sixth floor in an apartment building in a large city. The building has an elevator, but her apartment is at the end of a 100-foot long hallway. The laundry room is in the basement of the building. Zoe has been doing all her self-care and work tasks independently. She has had to stop going to her weekly luncheon with her woman friends because she is embarrassed about her decline in function and eating skills. She used to knit and quilt, but is no longer able to do these tasks either. She has always tried to maintain an upbeat attitude about her RA and hasn't let it keep her from doing her normal routine.

Zoe has had a recent severe exacerbation of her RA that required a visit to the doctor, who gave her steroids. She is quite weak, feels fatigued, and reports an overall aching and stiffness. Her physician feels that she needs a course of rehabilitation at home to address her deficits after this recent exacerbation.

Occupational Therapy Evaluation

Zoe has no deficits in vision, hearing, cognition, or perception. Sensation is impaired for light touch, sharp/dull, and hot/cold. Zoe is right-handed. Her left hand has a swan neck deformity of the left index finger, and there is fusiform swelling on both hands. She has bilateral ulnar deviation of 15°. Her hands have instability in the MCP and PIP joints with difficulty with tip-to-tip and lateral pinch with carpal subluxation in both hands. Her hand deformities are not fixed. She has decreased AROM in both hands with weakness of hand grasp. In addition, her shoulder AROM is flexion: 85° and abduction: 70°; bilaterally, PROM is WNL. Her gross-motor coordination is mildly impaired, and her hand dexterity is severely compromised. Her left hand is more severely impaired than her right.

She gets easily frustrated, and finds that she is always tired and feeling depressed about the change in her ability to do things. She has always been a "fighter," but is now beginning to feel that she doesn't have the energy to keep up the struggle.

Zoe is still independent in her ADLs, but now she only dresses in housecoats and slippers. Zoe says that it takes too much time and effort to dress in her nice clothes, but she laments this as well, because she won't go out unless she is "dressed nicely." She doesn't shower anymore because she can't turn the faucets on and off, so she takes a sponge bath daily in front of the sink. However, she doesn't feel that she really gets clean and this bothers her. She has difficulty holding her hairbrush and toothbrush, and can no longer wash, dry, or set her hair. Meal preparation, eating, and housekeeping chores are also getting difficult for Zoe. She has always been very fastidious about the way she keeps her home, and this is getting more difficult for her to maintain. She has difficulty cutting up her chicken so now she doesn't eat meat, except for ground beef, because it is too tough for her to cut. She has difficulty with opening containers, especially milk, orange juice, and cranberry juice. She has an old-fashioned hand can opener, which she has difficulty operating, but out of necessity she struggles with it. She continues to try and do her laundry, but the burden of carrying all her laundry and detergent down the hallway and to the laundry room in the basement is too much for her now. Zoe ambulates independently without devices, but walks slowly. Her dynamic balance is good. Static balance is normal.

She is pleased to have an occupational therapist come to her house to "help"her. Zoe's goals are to stay in her apartment, shower, and dress nicely, do her housekeeping, and resume going out to eat with "the girls."She spends her days watching TV because holding a book is tiring and turning pages of magazines is too difficult for her. She states she doesn't like TV that much, but it is all that she can do now.

QUESTIONS

Goals/Treatment Plan

1. Write a list of Zoe's strengths and deficits.

2. The HMO has given you six visits to treat Zoe, not including the evaluation visit. They are known for not giving more than their original number. How will you, in conjunction with Zoe, prioritize her needs?

3. If you are the OTR and giving this case to a COTA, how many visits a week would you recommend? Why?

4. Write your long- and short-term goals for Zoe.

5. Given that you only have six visits, how do you make sure Zoe is invested in OT treatment immediately?

Safety/Precautions

6. What are you safety concerns with Zoe?

7. What precautions must you be aware of with Zoe?

Self-Care/Work/Leisure

8. Zoe tells you how much she misses taking a shower. She just doesn't feel clean with a sponge bath. How will you address this issue?

9. Zoe wants to wash and dry/style her hair. How do you address this issue?

10. What techniques can you teach Zoe to help her with brushing and flossing her teeth?

11. Zoe has told you that she would like to figure out a way to wear her nice clothes (blouse, skirt, stockings, and bra). What do you anticipate may give her the greatest difficulty in dressing and undressing? Why? How will you address these issues in treatment?

12. Please describe at least two ways of teaching Zoe to put on and take off a back-fastening bra.

13. What can you suggest to assist Zoe with opening cartons, containers, and cans? If you are using adaptive equipment, how much will it cost?

14. Please describe the principles of energy conservation that you will teach Zoe.

15. What are the principles of joint protection that will help Zoe with her home management tasks (cleaning, laundry, meal preparation)?

NOTES

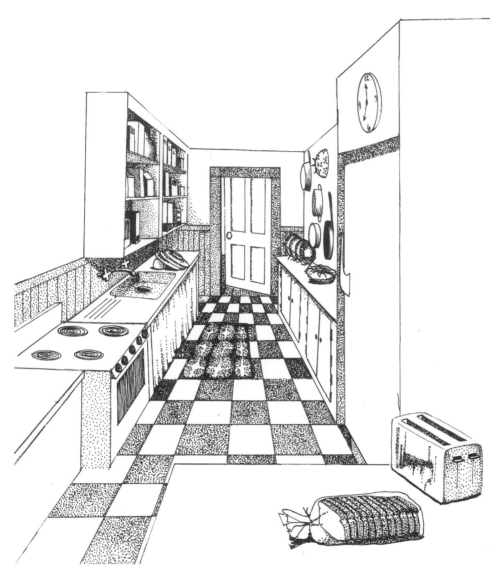

Figure 26-1.

16. What is a good way to teach Zoe to make her bed, including changing the sheets?

17. Zoe needs assistance with meal preparation. What techniques would you teach her for using the stove and oven safely, cutting vegetables, and lifting pots and pans?

18. From the history and evaluation, what are Zoe's leisure interests?

19. What will you address most immediately, given the six visits you have from her HMO?

Equipment/Adaptations

20. What types of adaptive equipment would you recommend to assist Zoe with her self-care tasks? Why? How much do they cost? Are any covered by insurance?

21. Using the diagram of Zoe's kitchen (Figure 26-1), how would you suggest that she rearrange her environment for greater efficiency?

22. What adaptive equipment would assist Zoe with meal preparation and why?

NOTES

23. What adaptive equipment would help Zoe resume reading again?

24. What ideas do you have to help Zoe with her other leisure interests?

Neuromusculoskeletal

25. Would you recommend splints for Zoe? Why and what type, specifically? Write a wearing schedule for Zoe to follow if you have suggested splints.

26. What types of exercise would you do with Zoe to improve her UE strength?

27. Write out a home exercise program for Zoe to follow between OT sessions.

28. Zoe has significantly decreased hand dexterity. What type of hand activities would you give Zoe to address this area?

29. Zoe is having difficulty preparing her insulin injections because of her hand deformities and weakness. How might you address this issue?

Psychosocial

30. You sense Zoe is discouraged with her situation and sees little hope in change occurring. How can you address this early in your treatment?

31. How do you think Zoe's OCD impacts her daily functioning? How do you see the relationship between her RA and OCD?

Patient/Family Education

32. You discover that Zoe doesn't have a good understanding of rheumatoid arthritis. What type of educational material can you give to Zoe? Find at least one website with information about RA and write the address. Describe why you feel this is a good resource for Zoe.

Situations

33. You are doing some hand exercises with Zoe and she complains of pain in her hands. What do you do?

34. You have discussed with Zoe how rearranging her kitchen will help her save energy, but she has not done anything after 2 weeks. What do you do?

35. You discover that Zoe has not been doing any of the exercises that you gave her. Instead, she is doing her own version. What do you do?

36. Zoe feels that she is entitled to all the services she needs for as long as she needs them. How do you explain to her that you cannot go over what the HMO has authorized, and that she needs to make the most of the time you have together?

37. When you arrive at Zoe's house one day, she is in the kitchen scrubbing the floor on her hands and knees. She is clearly in pain, but won't stop, even when you arrive. What do you do?

38. The nurse from the agency calls to ask you if you can help Zoe with her insulin injections. She is unable to manage the needle and vial safely to draw her medication. What recommendations would you make? Can you find adaptive equipment that Zoe could safely use?

NOTES

39. Zoe is very fastidious and has a routine for most activities that she rigidly adheres to. She doesn't follow any suggestions for energy conservation or joint protection because they vary from her rigid routine. How do you handle this?

Discharge Planning

40. Your six visits have ended, but Zoe's goals in relation to her self-care and home management tasks have not been reached. What type of recommendations can you make to Zoe so she can continue to work on these areas?

41. Zoe has gained AROM in her shoulders to 110°, but her endurance continues to be only fair. She has improved hand dexterity, and can now manage her insulin injections with adaptive equipment, but her hand function is still limited, according to her, because she cannot knit and quilt. Would you recommend outpatient therapy for Zoe? Why or why not?

NOTES

Chapter 27

Alice:
Multiple Sclerosis

Alice is a 51-year-old married Caucasian female with a diagnosis of multiple sclerosis (MS). She was diagnosed with MS 18 years ago. In addition, she also has a history of hypertension and recently has had several falls. Her doctor referred her to the Visiting Nurse Association (VNA). She had no hospitalization leading to her referral to the Home Health agency. Her doctor was concerned about the progression of the disease and of Alice's ability to manage safely in her home. Alice has been independent in home management and ADLs, but it was clear to her doctor that this was becoming more taxing for her to accomplish. He requested an OT and PT evaluation.

Alice lives with her husband in a two-story home in a rural area. Her husband, Jim, owns a large commercial painting company and works more than full-time. Alice retired 2 years ago from her position as a middle school teacher. She found the work too draining and physically demanding for her. She misses working with the children and being involved in the community. She has two grown daughters, both of whom live out of state. She talks with them infrequently on the phone.

Alice is a very independent woman with a strong personality. She talks loudly and comes across as very confident and sure of herself. She tends to minimize the impact her disease has had on her life and feels her doctor is "overreacting" in getting the VNA involved in her care. Her discharge plan is to stay at home.

Occupational Therapy Evaluation

The results of the occupational therapy evaluation indicate that Alice has no cognitive, perceptual, visual, or hearing deficits. She has decreased sensation to touch in her hands. She reports a "numb" feeling in both hands, but states it seems worse at some times more than others. She has limited AROM in both shoulders as a result of weakness. Her shoulder AROM is as follows: 100° flexion; 80° abduction; 20° extension; 35° external rotation; 75° internal rotation; 0° horizontal abduction; 55° horizontal adduction; 110° elbow flexion. All other AROM of UEs are WNL. She has decreased gross- and fine-motor coordination, especially as she becomes fatigued. Her ability to engage in a task before fatiguing is about 15 minutes. She ambulates with lofstrand crutches and appeared to put a lot of her body weight through her arms to the device. She has difficulty through all stages of the gait cycle and is unable to put her heels flat on the floor while she walks. She has no active dorsiflexion in either ankle. This appears to be due to increased tone in her LEs. She moves slowly because of limited AROM, strength, and hypertonicity in the hip, knee, and ankle flexors. She performs her transfers from bed and chair independently, albeit precariously. Her sitting balance is good; her standing balance is fair for static and poor for dynamic with the crutches.

She is able to dress herself except for donning and doffing shoes and socks. It takes her about 30 minutes to get dressed, and the procedure tires her out. She likes to dress nicely every day and wears classic style clothing—cardigan sweaters, crisp button-down shirts, pleated dress pants, and loafers. Presently, Alice is using a stall shower to bathe herself (Figure 27-1). She demonstrates shower transfers as follows: She leaves the crutches outside the shower stall, steps in over the lip of the shower, holding onto the shower faucet to pull herself in, and leans herself in the right corner to help her keep her balance. She gets out by reaching around the shower door for the sink to pull herself out. "I've been doing it like this for a long time . . . no problems!" Alice says.

Alice fatigues very quickly, but pushes herself to do as much as possible before "crashing for several hours on the couch." She does all the cooking and laundry, and says it sometimes takes her all day just to get the laundry

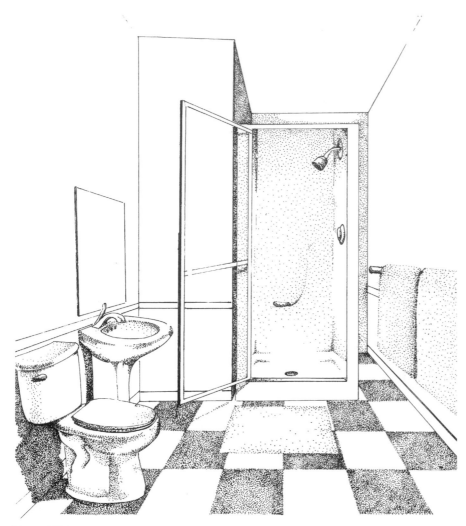

Figure 27-1.

done. The washer and dryer are in the basement, and the stairs leading down are very narrow. Alice refuses to demonstrate how she gets downstairs into the basement. "I manage!" she says.

Alice states she doesn't cook meals as elaborately as she used to do, but still makes them each night for her and her husband. Alice says she uses the oven "carefully." The stove is located in a part of the kitchen where it stands alone rather than as part of the counter. The refrigerator is located near the sink and counter. Alice's kitchen has a large table in the center of the room. There is no dining room in her home (Figure 27-2).

Her niece comes by weekly to vacuum the house for her. Alice insists on doing all the light cleaning herself. Her niece also takes her to the market weekly to food shop. Her husband is responsible for paying bills and money management. He also takes care of the home repairs and outside work.

Alice is skeptical about receiving occupational therapy and doesn't see how it applies to her. She is very clear about physical therapy, however, because she'd like to walk easier "without these bloody crutches!" Her goals are to "keep doing what I'm doing and not be a bother to Jim."

QUESTIONS

Goals/Treatment Plan

1. Explain occupational therapy to Alice in your own words.

2. What would you and Alice set as long-term goals?

NOTES

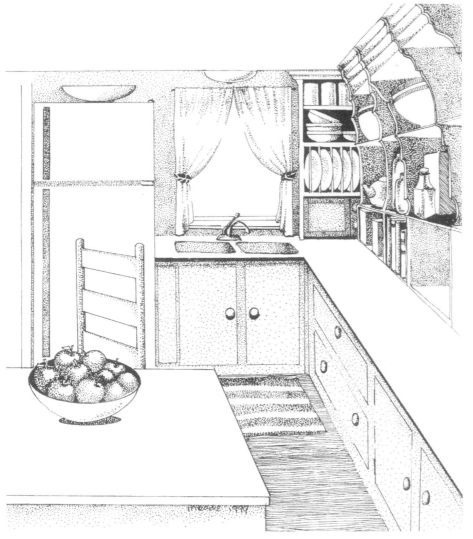

Figure 27-2.

3. What would you and Alice set as short-term goals for occupational therapy treatment?

4. Write out the treatment plan you would establish for Alice including frequency of visit.

Safety/Precautions

5. What safety issues do you see regarding Alice's present routines?

6. What things may Alice do differently to prevent any injury during her routines?

Self-Care/Work/Leisure

7. What changes could you suggest to make Alice's dressing routine easier?

8. What changes could you suggest for her bathing routine? (Refer to Figure 27-1.)

9. What techniques would you teach Alice to help her deal with her fatigue?

10. What alternative could you suggest to Alice if she feels too fatigued by late afternoon to prepare the evening meal?

NOTES

11. What could Alice do for meals if her symptoms are interfering with her ability to cook safely?

12. Alice loves to garden and misses being able to get out into her yard to tend to her flowers. She asks you for suggestions to help her resume her hobby.

13. Alice also loves to read while sitting in her reclining chair but gets tired from holding the newspaper open. She complains that she misses out on the news and asks if you have any suggestions.

Equipment/Adaptations

14. What adaptive equipment might Alice benefit from to increase her independence and safety at home?

15. Using a medical/therapy supply catalogue, determine the total costs of these items.

16. Prioritize the equipment you think she needs the most if she only has $200 to spend on supplies.

17. What could you do to help adapt her environment cost-free?

Neuromusculoskeletal

18. Write out a home exercise program for Alice.

19. How will you treat the sensory deficit in her hands?

Psychosocial

20. Why might Alice have been reluctant at first to engage in occupational therapy treatment? What functional activities could you recommend to work on UE strength and ROM?

Patient/Family Education

21. Alice's husband comes home one day during your session. He asks you what he can do to help Alice. She shouts out "Nothing! I'm fine. This is my problem." What do you tell him?

Situations

22. You arrive at Alice's house for a visit, and she calls for you to come in. As you enter the kitchen (Figure 27-2), you find Alice carrying a chicken potpie with one hand and trying to hold onto the counter for balance with the other. The food is obviously hot as the kitchen has a fresh-baked aroma. How do you address this safety concern with Alice? List several ways and her possible reactions to your comments.

23. Assume that after you mention this to her, she becomes defensive and tells you she's not a child. How do you deal with her feelings?

24. You arrive at Alice's home, and she is visibly shaken. She tells you she had fallen about 45 minutes ago and just got herself up onto the kitchen chair. She tells you she feels fine and she's just "mad at herself" for getting stuck between the counter and the kitchen table. She says, "It could happen to anyone!" What do you do? Alice tells you not to mention the fall to the PT or to her husband. What do you say?

25. You arrive at Alice's house for a scheduled visit. There is no answer at the door, and it is locked as always. She has never missed a visit before. You are worried she may have fallen and is unable to get to the door. What do you do?

26. Suppose you arrive at Alice's home and there is no answer when you knock, but the front door is unlocked. You are fearful she has fallen. Do you go in without being invited in? Please explain why or why not.

NOTES

27. You do go in and find Alice on the bathroom floor. She says she has pain in her shoulder and tells you to help her up. What do you do?

28. What could be done to improve Alice's safety during ambulation? What could be instituted so she could be safer while alone?

Discharge Planning

29. You have met all your goals with Alice and plan to discontinue occupational therapy. However, because of the nature of her disease, you know that it is likely that she will need further intervention. How do you explain to her the need to discontinue OT?

30. How can you be assured that she'll get the OT interventions needed once that situation arises?

NOTES

Chapter 28

Barb:
Left Cerebrovascular Accident, Right Hemiparesis, Expressive Aphasia

Barb is a 72-year-old Caucasian female with a diagnosis of left cerebrovascular accident (CVA) with subsequent right hemiparesis and expressive aphasia. She has secondary diagnoses of hypertension, a hysterectomy 12 years ago, and a history of transient ischemic attacks. She had never suffered a major stroke before this incident. Barb was hospitalized 2 months ago after her son brought her to the emergency room when he noticed she had a right-sided facial droop. She spent 2 weeks in the community hospital and then was transferred for a 6-week stay at an area rehabilitation hospital. She was discharged home from there.

Before her hospitalization, Barb lived alone in a small studio apartment (Figure 28-1) in a senior apartment complex. She has been widowed for 21 years and is used to taking care of herself and her own affairs. She retired 7 years ago from a position she had held for 32 years as a receptionist at a downtown law firm.

Barb has two sons, both of whom are married and living in nearby communities. She sees each of them about twice a month, as her sons both work long hours and are busy with their jobs and families. She has only one sibling, a sister, Beatrice, who lives in Florida. Barb visits her for the month of February each year.

Barb had been very active prior to the onset of her CVA. She went out with friends daily and was very active in the senior outings in her building. She always participated in the monthly bus trips they offered, her favorite being to the casino. She volunteered 2 hours a week at a soup kitchen where she served meals to the homeless. She walked indoors at the YMCA, approximately 2 miles three times a week. Occasionally, Barb would babysit for her grandchildren, ages 3 and 7, but reportedly expressed the sentiment "I'm too old for that...I've done my child raising already!" Barb never learned to drive, but did take public transportation everywhere she needed to go. She was independent in all of her daily tasks prior to the onset of the CVA.

Barb came home from the rehabilitation hospital reluctantly. Reportedly, she is unsure of her ability to manage at home and is afraid of failing and being put into a nursing home. However, her biggest concern is how to face her friends again. She is very embarrassed about her expressive aphasia and declined all of their visits and phone calls while she was in both hospitals. The discharge plan is for Barb to remain in her own apartment and manage safely with community health support services. She was referred to the Visiting Nurse Association for nursing, PT, OT, speech therapy, and home health aide services.

Occupational Therapy Evaluation

During her first visit from the occupational therapist, Barb is somewhat guarded. She becomes frustrated quickly regarding her speech and stops trying to answer questions when she can't get her point across after the second or third try. It is difficult to formally assess Barb's cognitive function because of her expressive aphasia. Her communication skills are limited by word-finding problems and difficulty articulating even one-word answers. Her vision, hearing, and sensation, however, are intact. She approaches new tasks in a slow, cautious, and disorganized manner. She has good judgment about her skills, but appears to have short retention and attention spans. She has difficulty with new learning and seems to prefer doing things "the old way."

Barb has approximately half of the normal ROM in her right shoulder. Her strength is obviously impaired and her gross- and fine-motor coordination is poor. She is unable to fully grasp or maintain a grasp on any items, rendering her right arm nonfunctional. She is able to oppose her thumb to the lateral side of the 2nd

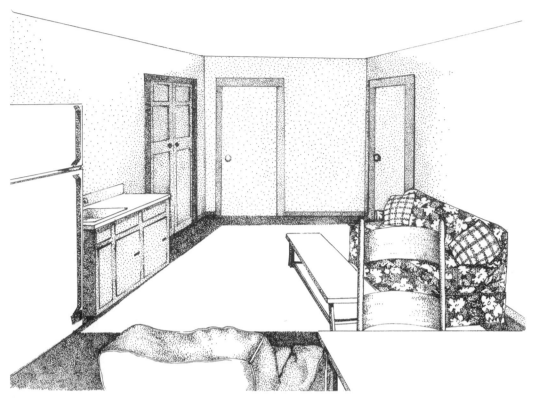

Figure 28-1.

and 3rd digits only. She is inconsistently able to extend all digits. Barb's right side is slightly hypotonic. Barb is right-hand dominant. She has pain in the right shoulder at the end ranges of all shoulder motions. She scores it a 4 on a scale of 1 to 10. She has slight edema in the right hand. She has no AROM deficits or strength deficits in her left UE.

Barb is able to ambulate independently with a small-based quad cane while wearing a right ankle-foot orthosis. She is able to independently transfer from bed and from chairs. She also transfers independently to/from the over-toilet commode. Her static balance is good; dynamic balance is fair. She has a shower seat and grab rails in her shower. She refuses to demonstrate the shower transfers and looks frightened at the suggestion.

Barb's couch is a pull-out bed. This is where she had been sleeping prior to the CVA. It appears that now Barb is sleeping on the couch without pulling out the bed. She is unable to pull out the bed or move the coffee table because of her limited strength and standing balance.

Barb is able to dress and sponge bathe herself in sitting without any adaptive equipment. She uses one-handed techniques for dressing herself. Barb confirms that she becomes tired easily during her morning routine, and it takes her much longer to get ready in the morning than before her stroke. She uses the microwave independently to heat precooked meals her sons bring for her. For convenience, her microwave is on the table where she eats. However, she is unable to demonstrate opening some of the containers her meals are in and has difficulty carrying food from the refrigerator to the microwave. She cannot open cans, bottles, or packages. Barb needs assistance for all home management tasks. She now has to rely on her sons to do all her shopping, laundry, and to pay her bills.

Barb says she wants to continue her work with occupational therapy. She says she wants to "be normal again."

QUESTIONS

Goal/Treatment Plan

1. Write out a problem list for Barb.

2. State how you would incorporate Barb's strengths to help her achieve her goals.

NOTES

3. What long-term goals would you and Barb set for her occupational therapy treatment?

4. What short-term goals would you and Barb set for occupational therapy?

5. Devise an occupational therapy treatment plan for Barb. Be sure to include frequency of treatment.

Safety/Precautions

6. What safety concerns do you have for Barb?

7. What could be done to ensure safety in Barb's environment?

Self-Care/Work/Leisure

8. After a few weeks, you are asked by the case managing nurse to do the home health aide (HHA) supervision visit. The HHA had been scheduled three times per week. The HHA tells you that Barb refuses showers. She only lets the HHA wash her hair in the sink. List three reasons why Barb might be refusing showers.

9. What do you suggest for each of these reasons?

10. Do you think Barb should continue to have a HHA three times/week? Please explain your answer.

11. How could you focus your treatment sessions so that Barb no longer needs the HHA?

12. Write out a plan to help Barb address her deficits in meal preparation.

13. What community resources may be helpful for Barb to manage her meals? Find the supports available in your community.

14. Barb still infrequently leaves the apartment during the daytime hours to get her mail. However, she will usually go out and do this around 9 P.M. List some reasons why she may do this.

15. Barb complains of back pain and gestures toward the couch. What can you suggest for her to do to be able to sleep on the couch as it was meant to be used?

Equipment/Adaptations

16. What adaptations may help Barb to be more independent? Be specific. Explain why these adaptations would be important.

17. What additional adaptive devices may be useful for her to maximize independence?

18. What problems may arise as you try to train Barb in adaptive equipment use?

Neuromusculoskeletal

19. What suggestions can you give Barb to manage the edema and pain in her right arm?

20. Why is it important to deal with both of these issues?

21. What could occur if the edema and pain issues aren't addressed?

22. Explain what occupational therapy treatment you would use to treat the hypotonicity in her right arm.

NOTES

23. Write out a home exercise program for Barb.

24. Barb asks why she has to do exercises. Explain to her why you are giving her exercises to do.

25. After 2 weeks, Barb shows improvement in the AROM of her right hand. She is able to maintain a grasp on large, lightweight items. What changes, if any, would you make in her treatment plan and/or goals? Why?

26. After one and a half months, Barb is able to use her hand as a gross assist. What tasks may she now be able to do that she couldn't do before?

Cognition/Perception

27. Given her cognitive status, how would you need to adapt your treatment sessions for Barb?

28. What could you do to be sure Barb was retaining new information?

Psychosocial

29. Even though she is unable to explain her feelings verbally, how might Barb express her feelings regarding the CVA?

30. What type of impact has the CVA had on Barb's family?

31. How has this changed their roles?

32. Barb declines engaging in social activities again. Explain the impact you feel this has on her and what could be done to address it.

Patient/Family Education

33. What type of education might benefit Barb's family in dealing with her diagnosis?

34. What are some of the ways you might provide education to Barb?

35. How could you utilize other team members to educate Barb and ensure carryover of treatment?

Situations

36. One day after 20 minutes of treatment, Barb becomes discouraged about her inability to communicate. She waves you off, gets up from the table, and walks away from you. How do you handle this?

37. How would you handle it if this behavior occurred for several sessions?

38. What could you do to improve your communication with Barb?

39. Barb's sister, Beatrice, wants her to come to visit for the month of February as she usually does. What are some questions/issues Barb should address **before** taking her trip?

40. After several months of therapy, Barb is able to use her right hand as a functional assist in daily tasks. She maintains the hope of full return to her right hand. She asks you if you think she'll be able to use the hand "normally" again. Write out what you would say in response.

41. Barb is upset after she returns from a doctor's appointment. He told her that her hand would never be normal. Barb is teary and upset. She tells you not to come anymore since it's not worth it. What do you do in this situation?

NOTES

Discharge Planning

42. At what point do you decide to discharge Barb from OT services? How do you know it is time for discharge?

43. Given that Barb doesn't want OT to end, how would you go about discharging her from service? Write a discharge note to Barb's doctor.

NOTES

Chapter 29

Charles:
Chronic Obstructive Pulmonary Disease

Charles is a 78-year-old African-American male with a diagnosis of chronic obstructive pulmonary disease, chronic renal failure, and depression. He requires 3 liters of oxygen via nasal canula. Charles smoked 1½ packs of cigarettes a day for 45 years and still sneaks a cigarette occasionally. He was hospitalized for 2 weeks with an acute exacerbation of his renal failure. During his hospitalization, various complications in his medical status occurred, and there was difficulty stabilizing his renal function. In addition, he became very depressed and despondent over his condition. He was discharged home from the hospital with home care services.

Prior to his hospitalization, Charles had been managing his self-care independently but slowly. His daughter, Clare, helps out with grocery shopping, laundry, and light home-making tasks (vacuuming and changing the beds). He spends his day watching TV and reading the newspapers. Occasionally, an old friend from his lodge drops by for a short visit.

Charles lives at home with his wife, Bessie, who has congestive heart disease and diabetes. They live on the first floor of a two-family house. Clare, her husband, and their two young children live on the second floor. Clare and her husband work full-time and their children are in daycare all day. Charles is retired from his job as a foreman in a factory that makes fiberglass insulation.

Charles has resigned himself to needing oxygen for the rest of his life, but won't go out in public because he feels that people are staring at him. He and his wife have separate bedrooms; she claims she can't sleep with the noise of the oxygen machine. Charles and his wife do not have a close relationship. He adores his daughter and grandchildren and loves to have them come visit often. His wife finds the noise from the young children more than she can stand in the apartment, and limits their visits to 15 minutes. Charles wishes he could go upstairs to spend more time with them but is unable because the oxygen tubing doesn't go far enough and he does not have the endurance to climb the stairs.

Charles does not want to go into a nursing home or assisted-living facility and wishes to stay at home. His wife is silent on the issue. In addition to occupational therapy, Charles is being seen by nursing to manage his renal failure and by physical therapy to address his endurance and functional mobility. He has a home health aide 5 days a week to assist with bathing and dressing.

Occupational Therapy Evaluation

Charles has no deficits in hearing or vision, except for glasses. His sensation is intact, and no perceptual deficits are present by observation during the evaluation. Cognition is mildly impaired for memory and judgment. He has AROM WFL, but has poor endurance, tolerating no more than 3 minutes of activity. During any activity, his oxygen saturation drops to 85% when at 2 liters, but at 3½ liters his oxygen saturation level remains in the low 90th percentile. He can transfer independently in and out of bed, and he spends his day in one chair in the living room. He has difficulty rising from the toilet and has to hold onto the towel rack across from the toilet to hoist himself up. He takes showers, but is so exhausted afterwards that he has to rest for an hour when he is done. Shaving is done standing at the sink. He dresses in T-shirts, slacks, and slippers. He does not wear socks or shoes because he can't bend over to get them on. He gets very fatigued with dressing as well. Throughout the ADL evaluation, Charles does not do any pursed lip breathing. Charles will get his own breakfast of coffee and cereal. His wife makes lunch, and his daughter will bring down dinner or make extra and put it in their freezer to be heated in the microwave.

Charles is very anxious and is afraid of getting out of breath with any activity. He has a very rigid routine and doesn't like to deviate from it. Little things are stressful for him, and his relationship with his wife also adds to his daily stress. He answers questions in a monotone and presents with a flat affect.

Charles is cooperative with his OT evaluation, but fearful of change. His goal is to be able to shower, shave, and dress without getting fatigued. He would like to be able to visit his daughter in her apartment, too.

QUESTIONS

Goals/Treatment Plan

1. What do you see as Charles' deficits and strengths?

2. What obstacles do you see in your OT treatment with Charles?

3. What are your long- and short-term goals for Charles?

4. What will be your frame of reference in working with Charles?

5. Describe your treatment methods for four of your short-term goals. Are they purposeful and functional?

6. What role will the COTA have in Charles' treatment?

Safety/Precautions

7. What are the important safety issues when working with someone who is using oxygen?

8. What precautions do you need to be aware of when working with Charles?

9. What is a safe range of oxygen saturation during activity?

Self-Care/Work/Leisure

10. Charles wishes to shower without fatigue. What techniques would you use to teach him to achieve this goal?

11. What techniques do you think would help Charles put on socks and shoes with laces?

12. Is bending over a good thing to encourage when working with individuals with COPD? Why or why not?

13. Is Charles shaving in the most energy-efficient manner? If not, what would you suggest to him?

14. It is important for Charles to be able to make his way safely around the kitchen for light meal preparation. What techniques will you teach Charles for meal preparation?

15. What do you identify as leisure interests for Charles? How might you address these interests?

Equipment/Adaptations

16. Figure 29-1 is a diagram of Charles' bedroom. How would you recommend that he rearrange it to provide maximum energy conservation in ADLs?

17. What adaptive equipment would you want to give to Charles to assist him with his bathing, dressing, and shaving routine? What is the cost of this equipment?

NOTES

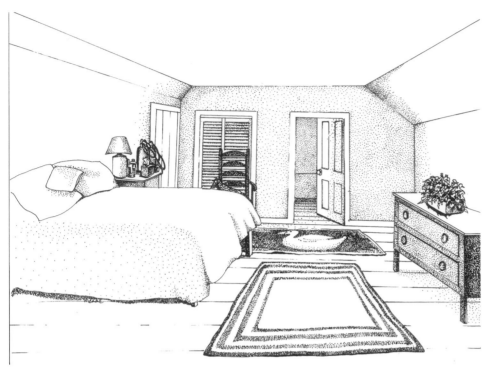

Figure 29-1.

18. What types of adaptations will you make in the bathroom to make it safe for Charles?

19. What changes in Charles' ADL routine would you suggest so that he does not get as fatigued as he currently does?

Neuromusculoskeletal

20. Because of his 2-week hospital stay and his general inactivity before that, Charles is quite deconditioned. Write out a home exercise program for Charles to increase his endurance.

21. Would it be appropriate to do UE strengthening exercises for Charles?

22. What type of breathing techniques do you teach Charles, and how would you incorporate breathing techniques into Charles' exercise program?

Cognition/Perception

23. Charles has difficulty in safety and judgment issues. How do you think this will affect him in his OT treatment?

24. What techniques will you use to teach Charles about the safety issues concerning his diagnosis? What safety issues should you be concerned about Charles having an understanding of?

Psychosocial

25. What impact do you think Charles' depression will have on his participation in his treatment?

26. What are some treatment activities that will address Charles' depression and anxiety?

NOTES

Situations

27. You are in the middle of an ADL treatment session with Charles when he begins to get short of breath; he wants to stop the treatment session and will not continue. What do you do?

28. In the above scenario, Charles has regained his breath, but still refuses to continue with the session. He tells you he just can't do it, and you notice his anxiety is very high. What do you do?

29. What techniques would help Charles to reduce his anxiety and stress? Is it the role of OT to instruct him in these techniques? How would you document this?

30. Charles is in the middle of an ADL treatment session. He is still having difficulty incorporating proper breathing techniques into his daily routine, and you need to remind him frequently. At one point, he stops and tells you he would rather be dead than to continue living like this. How do you respond to this?

Discharge Planning

31. Charles has reached most of his goals, but has plateaued at the level of minimum assist for lower body dressing. He continues to need oxygen at 2½ liters during all ADLs and reminders for proper breathing during activity. What type of discharge instructions do you write for him?

32. Given Charles' status above and his inconsistency with his home exercise program, would you recommend him for outpatient therapy? Why or why not?

NOTES

Chapter 30

Dimitre:
Right Fractured Radius and Ulna,
6 Weeks Post-Injury

Dimitre is a 92-year-old Russian man who lives alone. He fell in his bathroom and fractured his right distal radius and ulna. He called his neighbor, who drove him to the emergency room. X-rays revealed a clean fracture with no need of surgery to stabilize the fractures. His arm was placed in a full arm cast with elbow in flexion in the emergency room, and his neighbor drove him home. He has a history of non-insulin dependent diabetes, congestive heart failure, cataracts, and ETOH abuse. He did have his left cataract removed several years ago, but his right one cannot be removed because of macular degeneration in that eye.

Dimitre lives alone in his first-floor apartment. He is widowed with two sons, one who is in a nursing home with Parkinson's disease, and the second who passed away at the age of 70 from a heart attack. He had no other living family. He had been living alone and independently prior to his fall. He does not drive, but likes to walk daily, regardless of the weather. He goes to the neighborhood store to buy milk, vegetables, and fruit. Once every other week, a volunteer from senior services takes him to a large grocery store where he buys staples. Dimitre has a pet bird that he lets out of the cage daily. The bird is trained to go back into its cage when Dimitre tells it to. He is very fond of his bird. They have "conversations," and Dimitre calls the bird "his family."

Dimitre came to this country 20 years ago to be near his sons. He never really learned the language well. He lived with his son prior to his nursing home placement. Dimitre is not able to care for his son and feels very guilty that he cannot take care of him or see him often. The nursing home is too far to walk, and there is no public transportation to get there. Dimitre has to rely on a volunteer from senior services to take him there, but doctor appointments take priority, so he never knows when they will call him to offer the ride.

Dimitre is a fiercely independent man who lived through much in his Russian homeland. He does not like to ask for help, and he has a difficult time accepting help from others.

He is being seen in home care by nursing and occupational therapy. His right upper extremity cast has just been removed.

Occupational Therapy Evaluation

Dimitre's cognition is intact, except for decreased memory, which affects his ability to remember to take his medications. He has no significant perceptual deficits. He wears glasses, and his vision is poor in his right eye due to his cataract. Sensation in his hands is decreased for sharp/dull, and he complains of numbness and tingling in his right hand, especially his fingers.

He has strength in his left UE of 4/5 throughout. His right UE has 4/5 in shoulder movements, but 3+/5 in the elbow and hand and 3−/5 in his wrist. His has edema of the wrist and fingers, and he complains of pain with most wrist movements. He has AROM in his elbow of minus −25° extension; in his wrist of 20° flexion and 15° extension. His fingers are −1/3 of full ROM. His coordination is impaired for fine-motor and dexterity tasks with his right UE, but intact for the left UE. His gross-motor coordination is mildly impaired on the right UE due to his decreased elbow AROM; his left is WFL. Dimitre is right-handed.

Dimitre is independent in all transfers. He can shower with moderate assistance and dresses his upper and lower body with minimum assistance. Fasteners are difficult for him to do. He can't tie his shoes, and he requires minimum assistance to button his shirt and zip his slacks. Dimitre ambulates with a cane of his own making.

Prior to his fracture, he held this in his right hand. He has had difficulty with many of his home management tasks, including meal preparation, cleaning, and laundry. He is frustrated with himself and will not ask for more help from anyone, even though his neighbor has offered.

He looks forward to occupational therapy so that he can "get better." When asked for more specifics, he says he wants "to use his hand again like before."

QUESTIONS

Goals/Treatment Plan

1. Given Dimitre's goals, write a problem list and prioritize it from most important to least important.

2. What obstacles might there be to achieving his goals?

3. Please write long- and short-term goals addressing meal preparation.

4. Please write functional long- and short-term goals to address his UE status.

5. What frame of reference would you use to address the issues with his fractures? How will you address these goals in a functional manner and incorporate purposeful activity into your treatment session?

6. Given Dimitre's limited knowledge of English, how will you communicate with him?

Safety/Precautions

7. What safety issues do you want to be aware of when working with Dimitre? How will you explain these to Dimitre so that he understands them?

Self-Care/Work/Leisure

8. What are Dimitre's deficits in the occupational performance area of work? Can you make some assumptions about the difficulties he might have in areas that are not specifically mentioned in the evaluation?

9. Create a meal preparation treatment session for him that is culturally sensitive. State your goal, materials, and time frame.

10. How will you address Dimitre's bathing deficits?

11. How will you address Dimitre's dressing deficits?

Equipment/Adaptations

12. What, if any, adaptive equipment do you feel Dimitre might benefit from for his bathing and dressing? What is the cost of this equipment?

13. Dimitre's laundry room is in the basement. He usually carries his clothes down in a small wicker basket, but cannot grasp it well enough now to use it. What modifications can you think of to address this issue?

14. Dimitre likes to keep his electric bill down, so he uses very low wattage bulbs in his house and doesn't like to turn the lights on. You suspect this may have contributed to his fall. How will you approach Dimitre to encourage him to address these issues?

NOTES

Neuromusculoskeletal

15. Write a home exercise program for Dimitre to follow.

16. What functional activities can you do to increase Dimitre's AROM and strength in his right wrist and elbow?

17. Given his decreased hand dexterity and fine-motor coordination, write up four treatment activities that might address this area. Which ones are functional and/or purposeful?

18. Grade the above activities for improvement in his dexterity and fine-motor skills.

19. How will you address his decreased sensation?

20. Given that your home health agency has a very small budget for supplies and does not provide theraband, theraputty, or any other exercise equipment, what common household objects can you use for improving strength?

21. How will you address the edema in Dimitre's hand and wrist?

Cognition/Perception

22. Dimitre has a poor memory and forgets to take his medication, perform his daily exercises, and can't find where he has put commonly used items, like his eyeglasses, keys, and wallet. How can OT address these issues?

Psychosocial

23. Dimitre is fiercely independent and resists most of your ideas about help and changes to his routine and environment. How can you address these issues?

24. What aspects of Dimitre's cultural background are important for you to understand?

Patient/Family Education

25. Who are the supports that you identify for Dimitre? How can you incorporate them into your treatment planning?

26. What are some important education issues in this case?

27. Given Dimitre's memory deficits and cultural issues, how will you address patient education?

Situations

28. You have been starting off your treatment sessions with a few minutes of exercises. Today when you do this, Dimitre complains of pain in his wrist. You feel it and notice it is warm to touch and slightly swollen. What do you do and why?

29. What types of activities would you work on that do not exacerbate his wrist pain?

30. Dimitre wants to try cooking a complex Russian meal for you. It will take over an hour and a half to complete the activity. You have a productivity standard of six patients per day, and this will mean you see your last patient very late. How do you handle this situation?

NOTES

31. Dimitre's wrist has healed in a poorly aligned position. He complains of wrist pain when he wakes in the morning and of numbness and tingling in his hands. What do you think might be the cause of this, and what do you do?

Discharge Planning

32. Dimitre has achieved all but a few goals. He still does not have full AROM in his wrist and fingers, but they are now functional. Would you recommend outpatient therapy for him?

33. How would you arrange to get Dimitre to outpatient therapy?

NOTES

Part VIII

Inpatient Psychiatric Hospital

Chapter 31

Elizabeth:
Major Depression, Suicide Attempt

Elizabeth is a 25-year-old female with a diagnosis of major depression with suicide attempt by overdose of Acetametaphine with codeine. She was sent to the hospital emergency room from college health services, where her roommate had taken her when she started talking about killing herself. She had stopped eating and was having difficulty concentrating on her studies as well. Elizabeth is in her last year of law school. She had been doing well until she and her boyfriend of 4 years broke up. They met during their sophomore year at college and had been together ever since. Elizabeth assumed they would get married. They had applied to all the same law schools and decided which one to go to together. They did not live together, because Elizabeth felt that she wanted to wait until they got married. They were having a sexual relationship however. Law school was difficult for Elizabeth, and she had to spend more time in the law library than her boyfriend. Because of this, they didn't see each other as much as either would have liked. Elizabeth was surprised when he told her that he had met someone else whom he wanted to date and that he felt it would be better if they broke up. He said that he wanted to remain friends and that he just needed time to explore in order to find out if she was the one that he wanted to marry.

Elizabeth grew up in a large city as the youngest of three children. Her mother died from breast cancer when she was 13, and her father remarried 18 months later. Elizabeth did not get along with her stepmother and was thrilled to go as far away from her family as she could for college. Her father supports her during college, and she gets summer jobs to pay for books, clothes, and entertainment. Elizabeth has two older brothers to whom she is fairly close, but they live in different states from her and she talks to them by phone once a month. She usually hears from them by email once a week.

Prior to her hospitalization, Elizabeth had been living in an apartment with her roommate of 2 years. They share all the cooking and chores of the apartment, but each has a separate bedroom. She works hard at school and maintains a B average. She is looking forward to finishing and working in family law. Elizabeth is a hard-working, driven person. She feels that she has to prove to her older brothers and father that she is a capable person in her own right and that they don't have to protect her. She was very close to her mother, and her death was very difficult for her.

She is on the locked unit on suicide precautions. She is being seen by the milieu team: a social worker, psychiatric nurse, and occupational therapist, as well as her psychiatrist.

Occupational Therapy Evaluation

Elizabeth is evaluated by OT the morning after she was admitted from the emergency room. She appears disheveled; her hair is uncombed and her clothes are unkempt. Her affect is flat and she makes little eye contact. She speaks softly and looks down when she talks. Elizabeth has difficulty thinking of interests because everything that she thinks about are things that she and her boyfriend did together, and she starts to cry. She scored a 5.2 on the Allen's Cognitive Level. She mentions that they camped together and liked the outdoors, movies, and reading. She can't think of things she did by herself before she met him. She speaks about wanting to join her mother, "now that she has lost everything worthwhile in her life." She is on suicide precautions with checks every 15 minutes. Her expected length of stay is 2 weeks, with discharge expected back to her own apartment. While pessimistic about her ability to do so, Elizabeth is motivated by a desire to get out of the hospital in time to return to school to finish her last year with her class. Finals for the first semester are in 1 month, and her goal is to be able to take these with her classmates.

QUESTIONS

Goals/Treatment Plan

1. Write out a problem list based on Elizabeth's evaluation and history.

2. Given Elizabeth's goals, what are the long- and short-term goals you would set up with her?

3. What obstacles do you anticipate Elizabeth might face in reaching these goals in the expected time frame?

4. What strengths can you identify that might assist Elizabeth in reaching her goals?

5. What frame of reference will you use when working with Elizabeth?

Safety/Precautions

6. Given that Elizabeth is on suicide precautions, what safety issues do you have to be aware of during OT treatments?

Self-Care/Work/Leisure

7. Elizabeth had difficulty identifying leisure interests during the OT evaluation. How can you explore this with her, and what might you suggest, given what you know about her? Are there any additional assessments you might administer to assist Elizabeth in identifying leisure interests?

8. What treatment groups do you think Elizabeth might benefit from that would fit in with her treatment plan?

9. Elizabeth is determined to finish law school with her class, despite the fact that she is missing 2 weeks of classes and had been falling behind for 3 weeks prior to her hospitalization. How can you help her address this issue?

10. Elizabeth's roommate comes to visit and brings her some clothes and makeup. Elizabeth refuses to put on her makeup, saying "there is no one worth looking pretty for." She wears the same clothes that she came in with and refuses to change them. How can you and the team address this issue?

11. During a conversation with Elizabeth, you discover that she enjoys cooking gourmet meals. What can you do with this information? What if there is a kitchen on the unit? What if there is no kitchen on the unit?

Psychosocial

12. Elizabeth does not interact with other group members. She keeps to herself and speaks very softly. What types of group activities would encourage increased social interaction?

13. Elizabeth starts to cry at anything that reminds her of her boyfriend. This can be during groups, community meetings, or watching TV. It is especially disruptive during groups. How do you handle this when it occurs during your groups?

Patient/Family Education

14. What websites can you find that might be helpful to Elizabeth?

15. What types of education would you do with Elizabeth about her diagnosis and stress when she leaves the hospital?

NOTES

Situations

16. It is the second week of Elizabeth's hospitalization, and she has been showing signs of improving. You have just finished an art therapy group that required them to use scissors, and you find that there is a pair of scissors missing. Elizabeth left the room very quickly after the group ended, and you suspect she might have taken them. What do you do?

17. Continuing from the question above: You have talked to Elizabeth about the scissors, and she has flatly denied taking them. She gets angry at you and says she is going to report you for harassing her. You feel very confident that Elizabeth has the scissors. What do you do?

18. Elizabeth talks daily with her father, who wants her to come home for the rest of the semester. Elizabeth tells him she won't do this, but he keeps insisting. She tells you this and asks what she should do. She hasn't talked about this with any other team members. What do you do?

19. Elizabeth has been coming to life skills group every day for 1 week. Your goal is to have her start making choices about the tasks she wishes to complete and to do some problem-solving about this. She has been having a very difficult time making choices and keeps asking you to tell her what to do. How can you assist her in this area?

Discharge Planning

20. Elizabeth is ready to be discharged as planned. Write a discharge note to go to the university's health service.

NOTES

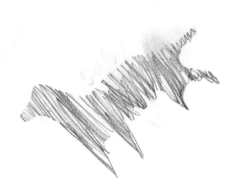

Chapter 32

Freddie:
Schizophrenia,
Paranoid Type with Acute Psychosis

Freddie is a 19-year-old Caucasian male with a diagnosis of paranoid schizophrenia with acute psychosis. Freddie has no other diagnoses in his medical history and has only been hospitalized once before because of his schizophrenia. Freddie lives with his mother in an apartment in the suburbs.

Freddie was admitted to the psychiatric unit from the emergency room of the hospital. His two older brothers, Jerry and Joey, brought him into the hospital at the request of their mother. Freddie had been becoming gradually more psychotic over the past 2 weeks. His symptoms cumulated with him locking himself in the bedroom over several days and refusing to let anyone in. Freddie believes his employer is trying to kill him. He had gathered multiple objects in his room to protect himself, including a knife, a baseball bat, and a hammer and refused to let his mother answer the telephone; he insisted they keep all the shades drawn and lights dimmed.

Freddie has been experiencing auditory hallucinations. He claims he can hear his deceased father telling him to "Watch out!" and "Look behind you!" Freddie says his father once told him to kill his employer, if needed, to protect himself. Freddie's brother Jerry convinced him to come out of his room to the car only by telling him that their father told Jerry to bring Freddie to a safer place. Once in the car, Jerry and Joey drove Freddie to the hospital. Freddie, suspicious and paranoid, tried to run away, but was tackled to the ground by his brothers. They got him to the hospital and luckily their mother had called ahead to notify Freddie's doctor of his arrival and the potential struggle once he arrived. Several orderlies were waiting for them and quickly restrained Freddie before he could run away.

Freddie's symptoms began after he was suspended from work. Freddie has been working at a distribution house where he loads boxed items into trucks. He had been an employee for only 3 months. Freddie reported that one of his co-workers told him to move boxes from the warehouse to the loading dock using the forklift. His co-worker gave him a quick demonstration and then left the area. Freddie attempted to move the boxes with the lift and instead ran them over, causing several thousand dollars worth of damage. Freddie did not have to pay the company back, but was suspended without pay for 2 days. This was 2½ weeks ago. Freddie has not returned to work since.

Freddie is admitted to the locked inpatient unit of the hospital. The plan is for Freddie to return to his home once he is stabilized. Freddie's psychiatrist is a physician on the unit and plans to follow his care. Freddie was hospitalized last year for 2 months after his first episode of schizophrenia; his doctor has been treating him since that time.

Occupational Therapy Evaluation

Freddie is seen by the occupational therapist after he has been on the unit for 1 day. Upon observing Freddie, he is somewhat unkempt; his clothes are wrinkled and dirty. His hands are also dirty, and he is unshaven. His hair is short but tousled and looks as though it needs to be washed. Freddie appears to be neglecting his basic self-care.

Upon approach, Freddie is guarded and minimally verbal. He makes no eye contact and looks down at the floor or wall during his meeting with the occupational therapist. He wrings his hands together constantly and rocks his body back and forth slightly in the chair. "I don't want to talk to you!" he barks loudly after introductions. He gets up, looks around, then returns and sits down in the same seat again. "Go away!" he says in a low, stern voice. "GO AWAY!" Freddie then leaves the group area for his room. The evaluation cannot be completed.

QUESTIONS

Goals/Treatment Plan

1. How do you help Freddie set goals if he is unable/unwilling to communicate with you at this time?

2. How do you attempt to complete the occupational therapy evaluation with Freddie?

3. What might you do to get the information needed for the evaluation, or do you have enough information already?

4. What are some problem areas that you can identify for Freddie?

5. What are Freddie's strengths?

6. Write out an occupational therapy treatment plan and goals for Freddie.

PG 435

Safety/Precautions

7. What are some safety concerns you have for Freddie?

8. What are some precautions the staff might make when approaching Freddie?

9. What would be the best way to approach Freddie?

10. What type of unit activities groups would <u>not</u> be appropriate for Freddie? Why?

11. What kind of unit activities groups would be appropriate for Freddie? Why?

Ch 10 pg 304

Self-Care/Work/Leisure

12. How might OT assist Freddie with improving his ability to perform his <u>ADLs</u>? Explain.

PG 502 Habit

13. How might OT assist Freddie with vocational <u>skills</u>? Explain.

Pg 515

14. How would you assess Freddie's leisure <u>interests</u>?

L 528

15. Assuming Freddie has deficits in all three areas, which would you focus on first and why?

ADL

16. Which would you focus on last and why?

Vocational

Ch 18 484

Equipment/Adaptations

17. What type of adaptations would need to be made to Freddie's environment to ensure his safety?

18. What type of adaptive equipment would Freddie need to enable him to be more independent in daily tasks?

Cognition/Perception

19. Describe the cognitive deficits Freddie's psychosis has caused.

20. Given what you know about Freddie, what level do you think he would be in according to the Allen's Level of Cognitive Disability? Why? *PG 84*

21. According to the Model of Human Occupation, where are Freddie's strengths and deficits?

PG 93

PG 606

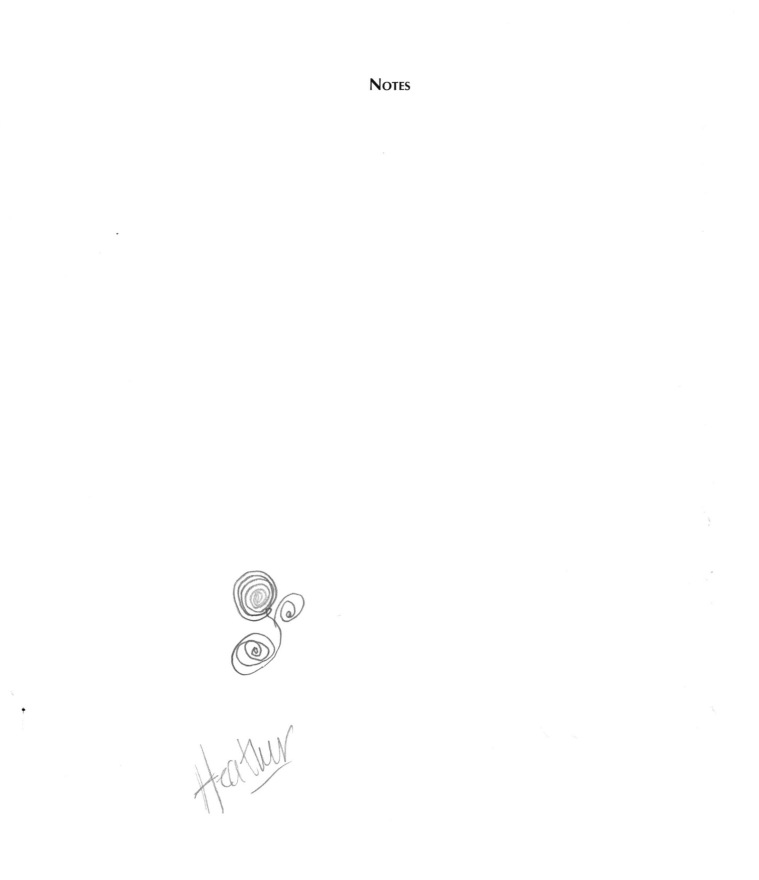

Psychosocial

22. What impact do you think Freddie's illness has had on his mother? On his brothers?

23. What impact do you think the hospitalization will have on Freddie once he is discharged?

24. What are some of the social skills that Freddie is presently unable to demonstrate?

25. How can the hospitalization and treatment help to change Freddie's psychological and social skills?

Situations

26. Freddie attends community meetings every day at the request of his doctor. What occupational therapy groups would you ask Freddie to attend? Why? groups ch 13

27. You are in cooking group and are about to make oatmeal cookies with three other patients. Freddie asks to join your group. This is his first time initiating involvement with others. What do you do and why?

28. You are in a community meeting and you notice Freddie shaking his head intermittently as if he is responding "no" to someone. What do you do?

29. Freddie frequently signs out the unit radio and listens to music quietly by himself at the end of the hall. How could you use this information to enhance Freddie's treatment plan?

30. Freddie continues to be withdrawn and isolated. How would you approach him to increase his socialization? Explain.

31. Freddie's doctor wants him to attend work task group. What questions would you need answered before you begin? Blue book - assessment

32. How would you set up Freddie's work station to simulate his work? What safety issues would you want to address before beginning the group?

Discharge Planning

33. Freddie is to be discharged from the inpatient unit to the day treatment hospital. Would you recommend occupational therapy for Freddie at the day hospital? Why?

34. What goals do you feel Freddie should meet before he is discharged from the hospital?

35. Write a discharge note for Freddie.

NOTES

Chapter 33

George:
Bipolar Disorder,
Manic Episode

George is a 37-year-old Caucasian man with a diagnosis of bipolar disorder, manic episode. George has a secondary diagnosis of alcohol and cocaine abuse and a past medical history of hospitalizations related to his substance abuse and his bipolar disorder. George is admitted to the locked inpatient treatment facility from the emergency room of another hospital.

George has reportedly become increasingly manic over the past 3 weeks. His symptoms include pressured speech, flight of ideas, grandiosity, and physical changes, such as voracious appetite, increased blood pressure and heart rate, and lack of sleep. George denies using any illegal substances. This is confirmed by his blood tests. George's wife reports he's been taking his medication, Lithium, sporadically for over a month.

George is a father of two boys, ages 10 and 8. He is currently separated from his wife, Nina, to whom he has been married for 12 years. He and Nina have been separated in the past, usually around the time the mania or the substance abuse begins. At his request, Nina is contacted when George is admitted to the hospital. She refuses to come to the hospital but does answer the psychiatrist's questions over the phone. "He stops taking his medication and gets crazy on me! I'm not letting the boys see it anymore. I'll do what I can to help, but I'm not going down there again!" she says.

George is an educated man with a master's degree in marketing and public relations. George has been trying to get his own business off the ground. Until 2 months ago, he had been working for an investment firm in the marketing department, but felt "confined by the rules of a large corporation." George had only been at this job for less than a year. He is very good at what he does, but his egotistical personality and his unreliability often result in conflicts with management. The pattern usually continues with George either quitting or getting fired. In the last instance, George quit his job with the plan of running his own business full-time rather than on a consulting basis. However, his own business is not doing very well, simply because he has not been able to stay focused on it long enough to make it run smoothly. Prior to the exacerbation of his illness, George had been working full-time and managing his home and own self independently. When he is not experiencing symptoms, he is described as very social and fun to be around.

The plan is for George to remain at the hospital until his symptoms are under control. The discharge plan is for George to return to the community. His wife makes it clear that he is not welcome back in their home as long as he is experiencing manic symptoms. She expresses that she might not let him back into their home at all. George is to be involved with all the disciplines on the unit including the psychiatrist, nursing, recreation, OT, pastoral counseling, and social work.

Occupational Therapy Evaluation

Upon approach, George is eager to talk with an occupational therapist. "I've been waiting for you to get to me! When can I start groups?" he shouts down the hall as the OT walks toward him. The therapist leads George into an evaluation room. The room has a small table and two chairs. There are large glass windows on either side of the door so staff can see in and patients can see out. During the evaluation, George has a difficult time remaining in his seat. He gets up and then sits down again frequently (Figure 33-1). When he is sitting, he is unable to sit still. He picks pieces of lint off the chair, kicks the table leg, and twists the phone cord until the receiver falls off the hook.

Figure 33-1.

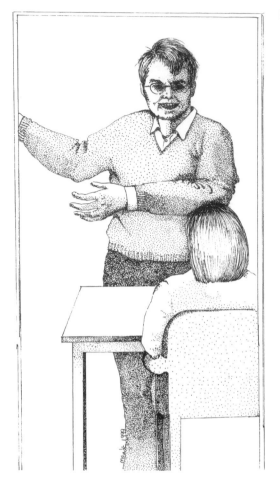

George is unable to stay focused on the conversation. His speech is pressured and tangential. His eyes dart about as he speaks, and he is unable to maintain eye contact for longer than a few seconds. His attention span is under a minute. George appears to have no visual or hearing deficits and in fact seems acutely aware of all the noises and sights around him, as he comments and yells out in response to every sound he hears. He notices every person who walks by the evaluation room and bellows out a greeting to them. Several times during the evaluation, he stands up at the table and yells over the therapist's head to someone out in the hallway (see Figure 33-1). He is unable to filter out external stimuli during the evaluation. He scores a 4.9 on the Allen's Cognitive Level test.

George appears to have no physical limitations. He ambulates independently with a quick cadence. As he walks, he runs his hands along the walls, possibly to take in more stimuli. The nurses say that he dressed himself this morning but refused to shower. He is clean-shaven, however. George claims he is independent in all work tasks, but this cannot be verified, as he is unable to attend long enough to complete the evaluation.

George responds to questions regarding his leisure time with answers like "What leisure time?" and "Leisure is my life!" When asked about attending programs on the unit and being involved with occupational therapy, George responds "I love occupational therapy!" When asked about his goals for occupational therapy treatment, his reply is "to make something for the kids in art class."

QUESTIONS

Goals/Treatment Plan

1. Review again the evaluation session with George. What could have been done to minimize his symptoms and further the evaluation process?

2. Write out a problem list for George.

NOTES

3. List George's strengths.

4. What goals would you set for occupational therapy treatment for George since he cannot set them for himself? What types of groups do you feel George would benefit from? Why?

5. What difficulties might you anticipate arising while working with George toward his goals?

6. How might you collaborate with other team members to assist in meeting these goals?

7. Write out a specific treatment plan including frequency.

Safety/Precautions

8. What are some safety issues that may arise while George is on the unit?

9. What are some things occupational therapy clinicians can do to minimize these safety risks during occupational therapy groups?

10. What types of treatment or groups would be unsafe for George at this time?

Self-Care/Work/ Leisure

11. How would you begin to address George's self-care deficits?

12. What type of treatment plan would you devise to focus on George's vocational issues?

13. How would you implement this treatment plan?

14. What role do you think leisure would have in George's treatment plan?

15. How important do you feel leisure is in his recovery? Why?

Equipment/Adaptations

16. What type of adaptations would need to be made for George to be successful in a group setting?

17. What type of adaptations would need to be made for George to be successful in a one-to-one meeting?

Cognition/Perception

18. According to the Model of Human Occupation (MOHO), what are George's strengths and deficits?

19. How would occupational therapy work within the MOHO framework to address his strengths and deficits?

20. What could you do to work on George's attention span?

Psychosocial

21. What impact has George's bipolar disorder had on his relationship with his family?

22. How might George feel toward his family after the manic symptoms have subsided? Why?

23. How has his illness affected his relationships at work?

24. What are some social skills George is presently unable to demonstrate?

Patient/Family Education

25. How could the treatment team involve George's family in his recovery?

26. At what point in his recovery do you think George would benefit from education regarding his disease?

Situations

27. You invite George to a group and he agrees to attend. However, he arrives at the group 15 minutes late. George insists you allow him in since you did invite him. What do you do?

28. George tells you it's his son's birthday and asks you to allow him to use the staff phone to call home. He tells you he asked the unit manager and she said it was all right. You can see that George is very anxious and he is shaking. What do you do?

29. You are in a group with George and he begins singing aloud. Some of the other patients don't seem to be bothered, while the one sitting next to him gets up and moves her seat. What do you do?

30. George requests a singing group to be held on the unit. The other patient with manic symptoms agrees that she would like to go to a group like that. What are your immediate thoughts on the idea? What is your response?

31. George signs himself up for a walk to the store with the community living skills group. George does not have privileges to leave the unit at this time. How could you involve George without him leaving the unit?

32. George seems to feel comfortable with you. He asks you if he could call you after he is discharged. How do you respond? How would this make you feel?

Discharge Planning

33. George is being discharged from the hospital. What changes might you expect in his behavior by the time he is ready for discharge?

34. George's wife decides she does not want him to return to their house after discharge. Do you think he is able to go home and live on his own? If not, what type of placement options would there be for him in the community?

35. George is to attend a day hospital program upon discharge from the inpatient facility. What would you expect the OT focus to be in that setting? What recommendations would you make for his OT treatment?

36. Write a discharge note for George.

NOTES

Chapter 34

Harold:
Poly-Substance Abuse

Harold is a 55-year-old Caucasian man who was admitted to the inpatient psychiatric unit of the veteran's administration hospital from the emergency room (ER). He was brought into the ER by police after getting into a fight at a local bar. Harold was treated for minor cuts and abrasions. The owner of the bar knows Harold well and did not want to press charges.

Harold has a history of alcohol and heroin abuse that goes back 32 years. He started using drugs when he was in Vietnam and became addicted to heroin and then cocaine. He has been living in his own home and rents out rooms to his friends, most of whom are his "drinking buddies" as well. He has not been able to hold a job for more than a few months due to his substance abuse. Harold has tried a variety of different jobs and has been through several work retraining programs. He did find that he likes working with computers; however, he was unable to retain any job in the highly competitive job market. He would end up getting drunk or high and not show up for work for a few days, neglecting to call in.

Harold finished college prior to enlisting in the army. His father had served in World War II, and he felt it was his duty to serve as well. Harold was married for 6 years after he returned from Vietnam, and he and his wife have one son. They divorced because of his substance abuse problem and his wife and son moved away; she did not want their son to be influenced by Harold. He has not seen his son since they moved away 27 years ago. Harold has two siblings, but has little contact with either of them. Both his parents are deceased.

Harold would rather have fun than be responsible. He is easily influenced by his friends to go out drinking or score some cocaine. His entire social circle is made up of people he either does cocaine with or drinks with. He does not have the ability to make his own decisions and stick to them.

He is admitted to the locked psychiatric unit for detoxification. He will be seen by the psychiatrist, occupational therapist, and psychiatric nurse. He will be incorporated into the milieu of the unit and expected to participate in group activities as determined by Harold and the team.

Occupational Therapy Evaluation

At the occupational therapy evaluation, Harold presents as disheveled in appearance. He does not have any clothes with him, so he is wearing a hospital johnnie, hospital robe, and slippers. He is unshaven, his hair is still matted with blood, and it is clear that he has not yet showered. When asked by the OT if he wishes to take some time to clean up before the interview he asks "What's the point?" He is administered an interest inventory and indicated interests in watching sports on TV and going to movies. He appears easily distracted, loses his train of thought easily, and needs to ask for questions to be repeated. When given a simple copying task, he has difficulty following directions. He cannot remember the events leading up to his hospitalization. When asked what a typical day was like, Harold cannot give any specific information. He says that he and his buddies just "kinda hang around all day and do whatever we feel like doing."

It is unclear if anyone in the household is responsible for grocery shopping, cleaning, or any other home-making tasks, though Harold does not appear malnourished.

Harold had to leave the occupational therapy evaluation before it was completed because he became very anxious and started to shake. It is unclear what his goals are and whether he is truly invested in his recovery process.

QUESTIONS

Goals/Treatment Plan

1. Write out a problem list based on Harold's history and OT evaluation.

2. What do you see as Harold's strengths and weaknesses? How would you go about completing the OT evaluation?

3. How would you engage Harold in identifying some goals for OT?

4. Harold does not understand what OT is and tells you he doesn't want another "job shrink." How do you explain occupational therapy's role in the psychiatric setting?

5. What are some long- and short-term goals for Harold?

6. What frame of reference will you use to achieve your goals, and why did you choose this one?

7. What obstacles do you anticipate Harold might have in achieving these goals?

Safety/Precautions

8. What safety issues do you have to be aware of in working with Harold?

9. What precautions do you have to be aware of in working with Harold?

Self-Care/Work/Leisure

10. Harold does not have any clothing in the hospital and does not seem to care about his appearance. He has not taken a shower or shaved in a few days. How can you address this issue with Harold? What would be the first task that you would try to have Harold work on, and why did you choose this task?

11. Harold has agreed to take a shower, but wants you to be there when he does it. How do you respond to this situation?

12. What groups would you recommend to address issues of home management tasks?

13. How will you assess Harold's skills at money management?

14. Harold claims he likes computers, but has not been able to keep a job because of his substance abuse. What are some of the skills that he needs in order to be a productive worker? How will OT address these?

15. Harold has very limited leisure interests as expressed in his interest checklist. How would you categorize his stated interests, and how would the two of you explore expanding his interests?

Cognition/Perception

16. Harold has a poor memory, time management skills, and problem-solving skills. What types of group activities might be beneficial for him?

17. How would you structure tasks so Harold could follow them?

18. Patients on the unit are responsible for getting to their assigned groups. However, despite a written schedule, Harold always forgets his groups. How can you address this issue?

NOTES

Psychosocial

19. What supports, if any, can you identify for Harold?

20. What social skills can you identify that Harold possesses? What social skills does Harold need to develop? How would you assist him with this?

Patient/Family Education

21. What type of education will you need to provide Harold?

22. What is the role of OT in educating Harold about his disease? In what ways can OT assist Harold in coping with his disease?

Situations

23. Harold is in group one day. You think you smell alcohol on his breath. You know that one of his friends from his home visited him earlier in the day. Do you confront Harold? If so, how, and what might his response be? If not, why not?

23a. If you choose not to confront Harold in the above situation, what impact might it have on his treatment?

24. Harold is in one of your groups. He is very disruptive, has a short attention span, and keeps talking out of turn. How do you handle this situation?

Discharge Planning

25. What type of setting do you think Harold would benefit from when he is discharged from the VA hospital? Why did you pick this setting?

26. Do you think Harold will need continued OT when he leaves the VA hospital? What do you think he should work on in OT?

27. Write a discharge note for Harold. Address it to the appropriate person if he is to continue in treatment.

NOTES

Chapter 35

Irene:
Post-Traumatic Stress Disorder

Irene is a 19-year-old Hispanic woman with a diagnosis of post-traumatic stress disorder. Irene has a secondary diagnosis of loss of peripheral vision in her left eye, which resulted from a childhood playground accident. She has no other diagnoses. Irene is admitted to the inpatient psychiatric unit from her doctor's office. It is a voluntary admission on an open unit.

Irene has been "haunted" by the recurring thoughts associated with a fire at her home, which took the lives of her mother and two young brothers. The loss of her family and home happened 14 months prior to her hospitalization. Irene had not been home at the time of the fire. She had been called in to work to fill in for another employee who had not reported for duty. Irene worked as an assistant manager for a large pharmacy chain that has stores open 24 hours. Upon leaving the store after midnight, Irene went out for pizza and then drove home. She drove down her street around 1:30 A.M. to see the "smoke and flames everywhere!" Her house was engulfed in flames. There were several fire engines and fire crews on the scene. Irene's two young brothers (ages 4 and 5) both burned to death in the fire. They were found huddled under the bed in their mother's room. Irene's mother was severely burned because she had remained in the house trying to find her sons. She died later that morning in the hospital.

Irene has persistently been experiencing thoughts of the tragedy both in dreams and while awake. Frequently, Irene reports "reliving" the experience at the sight or suggestion of fire. She reports physiologic reactivity such as sweating and shortness of breath whenever there is any reminder of the accident. Irene claims it will happen when someone lights a lighter or if she sees fire on television. Irene has also been experiencing symptoms of depression, insomnia, decreased concentration, and frequent crying episodes followed by emotional numbness. Irene's symptoms have interfered with all aspects of her life. She had been working part-time at the store, but has not been to work since the accident. Because of the nature of her work absences and since she had been a good employee for the past 3 years, the company intends to keep her job for her. Irene had been enrolled full-time in a bachelor's degree program with the intent of receiving her degree in business management. Irene is a sophomore, but has withdrawn from her classes. In addition, Irene declines spending time with her friends and chooses to spend most of her time alone. She speaks very little and avoids interaction with others.

Irene is currently living with her aunt and uncle. Her Aunt Marlene is her mother's sister. Marlene has told Irene she can stay indefinitely. There is plenty of room in the house, since all of Marlene's and Douglas' children have grown and moved away. Irene's father, who lives out of state, has offered that she could move in with him, but Irene has declined. The discharge plan is for Irene to return to living with her aunt and uncle and continue counseling and treatment on an outpatient basis. Her expected length of stay is 10 days.

Occupational Therapy Evaluation

Upon evaluation, Irene is cooperative and quiet. She appears to have no perceptual, hearing, or sensory deficits. She compensates easily for her loss of left peripheral vision. Irene has difficulty concentrating, which affects her short-term memory and immediate recall. She has a slightly delayed reaction when responding to open-ended questions, but quickly answers yes/no questions. Irene does not initiate conversation nor does she ask any questions.

Irene has no physical limitations nor any complaints of pain. She appears tired and lacks energy. She ambulates and transfers independently and easily. Irene is independent in her self-care as reported by the nurse and mental health worker. She is neat and groomed, wearing a simple sweatsuit and sneakers. "At least I can still do that for myself," she says. Irene reports no leisure activities or hobbies.

Irene says her goals for the hospitalization are to help her cope with her loss and get rid of the constant "dull ache" inside. Irene says she wants to go back to work and school someday, but seems fearful that will never happen. Irene's goals for occupational therapy are to be able to do "something" without crying. Irene cries several times during the evaluation even though she is asked no questions about the event or her family.

QUESTIONS

Goals/Treatment Plan

1. What goals would you and Irene set for her occupational therapy treatment?

2. What are some of the problem areas for Irene?

3. What are Irene's strengths?

4. How could Irene capitalize on her strengths to help her meet her goals?

5. Write out an occupational therapy treatment plan for Irene including frequency. What OT groups would you recommend Irene participate in?

Safety/Precautions

6. What are some things you should keep in mind given Irene's diagnosis and situation in regards to safety?

7. What type of unit activities might be too difficult for Irene to tolerate at this time? Explain.

Self-Care/Work/Leisure

8. Explain how you would assess Irene's home management skills.

9. What areas of home management would you anticipate Irene will have difficulty with given her symptoms and why?

10. How might you assess Irene's vocational skills and habits? Explain.

11. What could you do in occupational therapy to address Irene's lack of leisure skills?

12. Do you think it is appropriate to address leisure skills at this time with Irene?

Equipment/Adaptations

13. What type of adaptations might need to be made to Irene's environment to enable her to function better?

14. How might you adapt the following activities to enable Irene to perform them more easily?
    a. Reading a book
    b. Looking at a magazine
    c. Watching television
    d. Following the unit schedule

NOTES

Cognition/Perception

15. Describe the cognitive deficits Irene is experiencing due to her illness.

16. What day-to-day difficulties would you anticipate Irene would have given these cognitive deficits?

17. Would you expect that these deficits are temporary or permanent? Explain.

Psychosocial

18. Describe in detail the range of emotions that Irene might be feeling. Use yourself as an example.

19. What can be done on the unit to increase Irene's social interactions with others?

Patient/Family Education

20. What type of education would Irene's family need to help her through her trauma?

Situations

21. Irene has not attended any groups on the unit except the community meeting each morning. She tells you she does not want to go because she is sure she'll begin crying for "no reason." What do you say?

22. Irene's doctor asks if you could work with her around her job skills. How could you incorporate Irene's job tasks into the unit program?

23. Irene is in the day room with a new patient. The new patient asks Irene why she is there, and Irene's response is "because I'm crazy." How might you respond to Irene's answer? Why might Irene have responded like that?

24. Irene gets a card from her co-workers. "How will I face them when I leave here?" she asks. What do you say?

25. You are sitting with Irene and she asks you "Have you ever lost anyone?" What do you say?

Discharge Planning

26. Irene is to be discharged from the hospital. She will be seeing a psychiatrist weekly for counseling and monitoring of medication. She will not be receiving any other services, including occupational therapy. How could you help Irene to carryover what she has learned from occupational therapy at the hospital?

NOTES

Part IX

Psychiatric Day Hospital

Chapter 36

Jayna:
Borderline Personality Disorder

Jayna is a 24-year-old Caucasian woman with a diagnosis of borderline personality disorder. She has a history of depression, suicidal ideations and gestures, and alcohol abuse. Jayna is referred to the day program by her outpatient psychologist as a means for her to gain control over herself instead of having to be hospitalized. Jayna has a history of multiple inpatient hospitalizations. Her psychologist, Dr. Jansson, believes that Jayna prefers the inpatient hospital to the real world because of the secondary gains she gets from being admitted. Dr. Jansson feels that the hospital allows Jayna to escape her problems and provides her with an "excuse" for not having to deal with any of life's stressors. Jayna often asks to be hospitalized and when she is denied, she makes several suicidal gestures until she is admitted. Undoubtedly, she is in great emotional pain, but it has developed to the point that Jayna is in the hospital more often than she is out of the hospital.

Jayna's psychiatric history began when she was 16. She ran away from home and was found later by police in another city when she was arrested for stealing. The school psychologist had determined that Jayna needed counseling and connected her with a psychiatrist. Jayna "fired" several doctors over the years until she found Dr. Jansson. Even though she is frequently angry with Dr. Jansson, Jayna has kept working with her for the past 3 years. Jayna visits with Dr. Jansson twice per week.

Jayna is to attend the day program on the 3 days a week that she does not have an appointment with her doctor. Jayna has reluctantly agreed to attend the program and makes it clear to Dr. Jansson that it probably is not going to be helpful.

Jayna is plagued with feelings of uncertainty regarding her purpose in life and self-worth. She anguishes constantly about what she will do with her life and frequently begins things such as classes or jobs only to quit them soon after. She also longs for a companion and attempts to coerce men into intense relationships by using sex as a bargaining tool. Jayna's behavioral patterns include frequent episodes of intoxication and binge drinking. She will sometimes then engage in promiscuous sexual encounters with a man who she meets while drinking. Expecting a deep, meaningful relationship with the man, Jayna becomes irritable, angry, and sometimes violent if he does not return her intensity regarding the relationship. She has been physically injured several times by men after such an encounter. Jayna sometimes convinces the man to see her again with the promise of sex. Jayna alternates between feeling intense "love" for the man and bitter hatred. Eventually, a "dull void" overwhelms her and she often begins self-mutilating behavior such as burning herself or superficial scratching on her forearm. Soon afterward, she asks to go into the hospital.

Jayna lives with her mother and her mother's boyfriend. Her father left them when she was 12, and she has not heard from him since. Jayna's mother works and spends her free time gambling at the horse and dog track. Jayna says she "hates" Tom, her mother's boyfriend, and refuses to speak to him.

Jayna does not work. She has been unable to hold a job for more than a few weeks, either because "the boss is an ass" or the job is "boring as hell." Jayna has attempted college multiple times. She enrolled in several classes in psychology, sociology, and English at different schools. She completed only two classes and either had to drop out because of a hospitalization or just "lost interest" and never went back to the school.

Occupational Therapy Evaluation

Jayna is seen for an occupational therapy evaluation on her first day at the program. She is familiar with the schedule and the routine as she has attended this program twice before. Jayna presents as very neatly groomed and somewhat provocatively dressed, wearing a tight fitting mini-dress and spiked high heels. Throughout the evaluation, Jayna asks questions about the staff members and patients who attended in the past. She makes comments under her breath regarding the appearance of others as they walk past the room. She needs to be refocused frequently.

Jayna appears to have no cognitive, visual, hearing, sensory, or perceptual deficits. She has no limitations in her physical status, no complaints of pain, and no edema or skin changes. She reports continued independence in her ADLs and IADLs at home. She reports that her duties at home are to make her own meals, clean her own room, and care for her laundry. Tom pays all the bills and her mother does all the grocery shopping. Jayna does not drive; she takes the bus to get around in the community. She reports no difficulty in completing any of these tasks. Annoyed, she states she reached the day program on the bus that morning without help. When asked about how she spends her free time, Jayna laughs and says "Sex! How about you?" Jayna agrees to attend groups but says she doesn't need any occupational therapy. "I know how to bake brownies already," she laughs. Her goal of attending the day program is simply to keep a deal with Dr. Jansson and be finished with it as soon as possible.

QUESTIONS

Goals/Treatment Plan

1. Even though Jayna does not want to participate in individual occupational therapy, what goals would you set with her for group treatment?

2. What might you say to Jayna in response to her comment about not needing occupational therapy?

3. What are some problem areas for Jayna?

4. What are Jayna's strengths?

5. How might her strengths be utilized to help her participate in the program more actively?

6. Write out a treatment plan for Jayna. Be specific.

Safety/Precautions

7. What would be some of the safety concerns regarding Jayna as she attends the day program?

8. What type of precautions would the staff need to take to ensure her safety?

9. What are some of the safety concerns for Jayna outside of the day program?

10. What can be done to increase her safety outside of the program?

Self-Care/Work/Leisure

11. Given that Jayna has skill deficits in the areas of both work and leisure, which one would you choose to address first and why?

12. Explain how you would go about implementing your treatment plan.

Equipment/Adaptations

13. What type of adaptations might be made in regards to interactions with Jayna to promote more positive relationships with others?

NOTES

Psychosocial

14. Why might Jayna be feeling and behaving this way toward attending the day program?

15. What type of positive outcome can be expected from attendance at the day program?

Patient/Family Education

16. Jayna does not want her mother involved in her treatment. What type of family education can be done in this circumstance?

Situations

17. You are beginning a cooking group and Jayna passes by. She is not scheduled to attend but asks if she can participate because she has "nothing else to do and this stuff is easy!" What do you say and do?

18. You are leading a group that is sitting in a circle. Jayna is wearing a skirt and is sitting with her legs open so that you can see up her skirt. There are several male patients staring her way. What do you do?

19. What do you imagine Jayna's reaction would be to your response in the situation above?

20. Jayna is outside smoking a cigarette after lunch. You are inside the building and see her through the window. She pulls up her sleeve and presses the cigarette head against her forearm. What do you do?

21. What might the policy at the day program be to deal with self-mutilating behavior?

22. You overhear Jayna and a male patient planning on meeting after the program for a drink. Do you intervene? Why or why not?

23. What could be the consequences of intervening in Jayna's personal conversations? What could be the consequences of not intervening? Explain.

24. Jayna is talking with you during free time after lunch. She tells you about her last boyfriend and their relationship. She then asks you about your present relationship. What do you say?

25. Why might you want to share some information with Jayna about yourself? Why might you not want to share with her? Explain. What information about yourself would it be appropriate to share with Jayna?

26. It is time to begin group, and Jayna is obviously angry with one of the other female patients. She calls her a "bitch" and says she is not sitting next to her. How do you respond?

27. How do you proceed with the group given Jayna's obvious anger and how much it has unnerved the other members?

Discharge Planning

28. After 3 weeks, Jayna appears to be less irritable and anxious. She is interacting more positively with staff and patients. Dr. Jansson is pleased with how she is doing and hospitalization seems unnecessary now. In your opinion, should day hospital be terminated because the goals were met or should she continue because she is doing well? Explain your rationale for either decision.

NOTES

Chapter 37

Kara:
Anorexia Nervosa

Kara is a 22-year-old Caucasian woman with a diagnosis of anorexia nervosa. Kara also has recently been diagnosed with hypotension, malnutrition, and amenorrhea. Kara is scheduled to attend day hospital 5 days a week. She had been hospitalized 3 weeks ago on the acute medical floor of the hospital to treat her physical symptoms. Once she was medically stabilized, approximately 5 days after admission, she was transferred to the psychiatric unit where she had been until her discharge home 3 days ago.

Kara was diagnosed with anorexia nervosa when she was 17 years old. She was hospitalized once before when she was about to turn 18. Her parents forced her into the hospitalization because she had lost such a large amount of weight and was so sick at the time. Kara has been seeing a therapist on a regular basis since then. She has enrolled in college in a nursing program and did fairly well her first year. She initially had wanted to live on-campus, but her parents had not allowed it for fear that she would not take care of herself and become ill again. By Kara's third year, her symptoms seemed to be under control, and she begged her parents to allow her to live on-campus for her last year. The college is 20 minutes away from her home, and her parents reluctantly agreed. Kara is now about to complete her fourth year and is contemplating continuing on to graduate school to earn her degree as a nurse practitioner. Midterm exams were only 2 weeks away when Kara was hospitalized.

Kara had been losing more and more weight since she began living on-campus. She avoided coming home to visit her parents and once even hid from them when they tried to visit her at school. She made up excuses why she couldn't come home for a visit and purposely called them when she knew they would not be home so she could just leave a message and not have to answer any of their questions.

Her weight dropped from 119 pounds to 86 pounds. Kara is 5'9" and was too thin before she moved on-campus. She collapsed in the bathroom after a hot shower and was brought to the emergency room at the city hospital. Her parents were notified immediately, and they insisted she be treated again for the physical symptoms and anorexia.

Kara's parents are very loving and concerned. They tried to understand her disorder but truly do not. Kara is the oldest of three children. She has two younger sisters, neither of whom exhibit any psychological disorders. Kara is basically a quiet young woman with a few close friends. She is not much for crowds and tends to choose keeping to herself rather than going with the other girls to "hang out." Kara had a few non-serious boyfriends in high school and has only dated occasionally during college. She usually prefers to double date with her friends than go out alone with a man. Kara reports having no hobbies and no leisure time except for studying with classmates.

Kara does not work while she attends college. She does work during the summers at a day camp for disabled children. She has been doing that since she was 16 and loves having an impact on the children. Several of them write her letters during the school year to keep her abreast of what is happening with them. She enjoys receiving these letters very much and refers to the children as "my kids." Kara reports that one of the few times she stops her studies is to respond to their letters.

Kara is to attend the day program for full days to start and then switch to a schedule that will allow her to attend her classes. Kara wants to go right back to school after discharge from the hospital. Her parents forbid her to return and have moved her back home from the dorm. They will not allow her to live on-campus any longer and have cancelled her renewal for room and board for the spring semester. They are afraid to let her return to classes at all.

Occupational Therapy Evaluation

Kara is seen for an occupational therapy evaluation the afternoon of her first day at the day program. Kara is very serious throughout the evaluation. She rarely smiles or relaxes. She exhibits no cognitive, visual, perceptual, sensory, or hearing deficits. Kara does have an altered "perception" of her size, however. This is not due to a perceptual deficit but to her faulty belief system about herself in relation to others. Kara truly believes she is overweight and speaks of it occasionally during the evaluation.

Kara has no physical limitations as far as AROM, strength, or coordination, but does report fatiguing easily and needing to nap frequently. Kara has no complaints of pain, edema, or skin changes. She has no limitations in mobility or ADLs.

Kara reports difficulty concentrating and states she is having trouble staying focused on a subject matter and learning new material. She says she feels like she hasn't even gone to school this past semester and can barely remember anything that was taught. She claims she went to classes, took the tests and did fairly well, but cannot recall any of the information at this point. This revelation causes her a great deal of anxiety because she needs to retain the information for the nursing certification exam next year in order to get her nursing license and get a job.

Kara is eager to work with OT if it will help her to improve her concentration level and ability to learn. She says she wants to be able to think about something else beside herself all the time. Kara admits to feeling "bad" about focusing on herself so much but feels she cannot stop.

QUESTIONS

Goals/Treatment Plan

1. What are some of the problem areas for Kara?

2. What are Kara's strengths?

3. Would you set a goal for Kara that involved her symptoms of anorexia, such as eating regular meals? Explain why or why not.

4. How might Kara be able to capitalize on her strengths to help her meet her goals?

5. Write out an occupational therapy treatment plan for Kara including frequency.

6. What specific occupational therapy goals will you help Kara set for herself?

Safety/Precautions

7. What are some safety concerns you have for Kara?

8. What are some things the staff at the day program might do collaboratively to maintain Kara's safety during her participation in the program?

9. What are some things you could recommend for her family to do to maintain her safety at home?

Self-Care/Work/Leisure

10. How would you address Kara's work skill goals? Explain in detail.

11. Would you incorporate the development of leisure skills into Kara's treatment plan? Why or why not?

NOTES

Equipment/Adaptations

12. What adaptations to the environment might be helpful for Kara to reach her goals? Explain.

13. What adaptations to her routine might be helpful for Kara to reach her goals?

Psychosocial

14. Describe the impact hospitalization has had on Kara emotionally, socially, and functionally.

15. Describe the behavioral impact it has had on her family.

Cognition/Perception

16. What strategies could you use to help increase Kara's attention span and level of concentration?

Patient/Family Education

17. What specific education would benefit Kara as she deals with her illness?

18. What type of education would benefit Kara's parents in supporting her through her recovery?

Situations

19. Kara does not show up for the day program 2 days in a row. What course of action should be taken?

20. Kara tells you she can concentrate much better now. How could you assess that?

21. You notice Kara throwing her food away at lunch. What do you do?

22. Kara comes to you, crying, and tells you her parents want her to drop out of nursing school. How do you respond?

23. While in group, Kara begins talking off the subject about how unhealthy fried foods are for you. It takes you several attempts to redirect her to the topic. What might you assume about Kara from her verbal tangent?

Discharge Planning

24. At what point do you think Kara would be ready for discharge from the day program?

25. What things would need to be in place or established for Kara to transition easily from the day program?

26. What type of education would her family need to assist her in this transition?

27. What type of follow-up care do you think Kara should have? Why?

NOTES

Chapter 38

Leo:
Schizoaffective Disorder, Depressive Type

Leo is a 31-year-old African-American male with a diagnosis of schizoaffective disorder, depressive type. Leo also has a secondary diagnosis of cannabis abuse. Leo is scheduled for the day program to assist in his transition from the acute care hospital back to the community and his job. Leo was hospitalized for a little more than 3 weeks with symptoms of auditory hallucinations, withdrawal and isolation, hypersomnia, and psychomotor retardation. Leo's hallucinations cleared, but he still exhibits the other symptoms, only to a lesser degree.

Leo has had multiple hospitalizations because of his schizoaffective disorder. Sometimes stressors in his life precipitate his hospitalizations, and other times he simply stops taking his medications. Occasionally, the onset of the acute symptoms of his illness do not appear linked to any factor at all. This is one of those times.

Leo was admitted to the hospital at the request of his case manager after several weeks of auditory hallucinations, which included voices talking about him negatively, sirens, and loud music. Leo became depressed when the voices spoke badly of him and began to sleep more, eat less, and grow increasingly isolative. The staff from the group home noticed his behavior changes and notified Leo's case manager, who, in turn, called his psychiatrist. Leo's doctor recommended his admission.

Leo's case manager, Amelda, has been working with him for 7 years. Leo trusts both her and his psychiatrist, Dr. Ramkasoon, and rarely disagrees with what either of them recommend. Leo does not like to go to the hospital, but he dislikes the auditory hallucinations even more.

Leo lives in a group home with three other men with similar diagnoses. Leo has been living there for several years. Amelda arranged it for him because his situation at home seemed to be too stressful and unhealthy for him. Leo's parents are divorced. Leo's father is schizophrenic and is occasionally found wandering and sleeping on the streets. Though not homeless, Leo's father often leaves his rooming house to later be picked up by the police for sleeping on other people's property. Leo's mother drinks heavily and regularly. She lets Leo stay at her house when she is sober. Otherwise, she makes Leo stay out in the garage. Leo has only one sibling, a sister, who is not involved with the family at all.

Leo does well at the group home. He does his own care with occasional reminders and participates in the chores around the house. Leo is responsible for setting and clearing the table and taking out the trash weekly.

Leo works approximately 8 to 10 hours a week with a cleaning company that contracts to clean offices at night. The supervisor picks Leo up on Tuesday nights at 9 P.M. and drives with him and another employee to the one or two locations that need service that night. The men work until the jobs are finished and the supervisor drives Leo home. That is the only night Leo works. Many Tuesdays, the supervisor has to wake Leo up to get him to work, but Leo has never refused. He has had this job for the past 8 months and appeared committed to keeping it. His supervisor, Scott, feels that even though Leo works slowly, he is a good employee and more reliable than most.

Leo is to attend the day program 5 full days a week. The plan is for him use the program supports to transition back to work. His doctor anticipates that Leo will only need the program for 2 weeks, maybe less. Leo is scheduled for an occupational therapy evaluation on his first day at the program.

Occupational Therapy Evaluation

Upon evaluation, Leo presents as withdrawn and minimally interactive. He is appropriately groomed and dressed. He does speak when spoken to, but answers in one- or two-word sentences. There is a delayed response when he answers and his speech is slow and labored. He rarely makes eye contact and stares down at his shoes throughout most of the evaluation.

Leo does not appear to have any visual or hearing deficits. He exhibits decreased problem-solving, short-term memory, attention span, and immediate recall. He also shows decreased organizational skills. He does not have any apparent sensory or perceptual deficits.

Leo's posture is slightly kyphotic, his hips in a posterior tilt, and he shuffles a bit when he ambulates. His ambulation is slow but he has no balance problems. His AROM and strength are WFL, but his coordination is slow and dexterity is impaired bilaterally. Leo says, "I feel stiff. I can't move right," when asked to perform simple manual tasks. He reports doing his own self-care and nods yes when asked if it takes longer than it used to. He shakes his head no when asked if he has resumed his chores at the group home. Leo states he has no pain. He also has no edema or skin changes.

Leo says he likes his work and wants to get back to it. He likes his group home and the people he lives with. He says he spends most of his free time watching TV, sleeping, or walking around the neighborhood because "I like being alone," he says.

Leo agrees to participate fully in the schedule at the day program. He is concerned about it interfering with his appointments with Dr. Ramkasoon, and is reassured that those appointments take precedence over the groups at the day program. Leo has participated in OT in the past and is vaguely familiar with its purpose. He says his goals for OT are to get back to work and feel better.

Questions

Goals/Treatment Plan

1. What are some problem areas for Leo?

2. What are Leo's strengths?

3. What specific goals for occupational therapy would you help Leo set for himself?

4. How might Leo utilize those strengths to achieve his goals?

5. Write out an occupational therapy treatment plan for Leo including frequency. What groups would you involve Leo in?

Safety/Precautions

6. What might be some safety concerns during Leo's attendance at the day program?

7. What type of precautions might the staff take to ensure Leo's safety while participating at the day program? At the group home?

Self-Care/Work/Leisure

8. What type of intervention might be beneficial for Leo to be able to perform his ADLs with greater ease and speed?

9. How could you assess if this intervention is working?

10. What types of interventions are needed for Leo to meet his goal of returning to work? How would occupational therapy be directly involved in this process?

11. How would you set up a work skills evaluation for Leo to determine his readiness to return to work?

NOTES

12. Does Leo have adequate leisure activities in his life? Please explain your answer.

13. How might Leo explain to his supervisor why he has missed so much work?

Equipment/Adaptations

14. What type of environmental adaptations might help Leo achieve his goals? Explain.

15. What type of adaptations to Leo's daily routine might make things easier for him to accomplish tasks in less time?

16. What type of adaptations might be necessary to Leo's work routine? What could be reasonably expected of his supervisor to accommodate?

Neuromusculoskeletal

17. What types of program activities might be difficult for Leo given his physical status?

18. What specifically would you recommend to deal with his dexterity and coordination deficits?

19. How could you ensure carryover of these recommendations for Leo when he is not at the program?

Cognition/Perception

20. Explain how you will address Leo's cognitive deficits.

Psychosocial

21. How might Leo feel about having to be hospitalized again this time? Explain why you answered as you did.

22. What impact do you think Leo's family has had on his life?

Situations

23. Dr. Ramkasoon asks you to work one on one with Leo on his vocational readiness. What will you do to address Leo's work skill deficits? Are there any formal assessments to address this performance area?

24. Dr. Ramkasoon also asks you to write up a protocol about how you assess work readiness so that he may better understand the process for future patients. Write an outline of what you would give him.

25. You are helping Leo review his schedule for the week. He cannot follow it and appears to "shut down" when presented with too much information at once. How can you present Leo's schedule to him in a manner that he can understand?

26. To help prepare him for resuming chores at his home, Leo agrees to clear the table after lunch. After his first day, you notice he has forgotten several empty glasses on the table. Why might this have happened? How could you use this opportunity to assess Leo's skills? How do you use this information in your next session with Leo?

27. The director at the group home calls asking for some exercises for Leo to do at home so he won't be so "zombie-like." However, Leo tells you he doesn't like exercise and won't do them. What activities can you suggest that would incorporate movement into Leo's daily routine without it feeling like exercise?

Short memory — Tv/Movie memory

attention span —

problem solving — puzzles ●

organization — time management

Calenders & ~~planning~~ planner

Short term memory group. for memory / attention span

Time management group for problem solving / organization

28. Leo's supervisor, Scott, calls the day program wondering how he is doing and when he'll be back to work. You feel Leo has shown much improvement and know the plan is for him to return in 1 week. What do you say to Scott? What do you need to do before you discuss Leo's status with Scott?

Discharge Planning

29. From an occupational therapy perspective, what objective information will tell you when Leo is ready to leave the day program?

NOTES

Chapter 39

Maura:
AIDS-Related Dementia

Maura is a 41-year-old African-American female who attends a day hospital community program 3 days a week. She has a diagnosis of AIDS-related dementia. Maura contracted HIV by intravenous drug use. She is currently clean of drugs and has been for 3 years. She converted from HIV to AIDS 2 years ago, and the progression of her disease has been rapid. She has been coming to the day program for 6 months, but her dementia has gotten worse and the staff is looking for assistance with how to handle her.

Maura lives at home with her 75- and 78-year-old parents. They have been helping her, but her dementia has become worse, and they also need guidance as to how to handle her at home. Maura has three children ages 21, 22, and 24. One of her daughters is a drug addict, her son is in prison, and the younger daughter lived in foster care most of her life and wants little to do with her mother.

Maura is on welfare and has never held a job. She has been in and out of detoxification centers and had lived in a homeless shelter before her parents finally agreed to take her in after her AIDS diagnosis.

Maura is friendly and enjoys the people at the day program. She has a sarcastic sense of humor and has offended a few clients in the past. She interacts during groups, but likes to spend time alone listening to music on her Walkman. She gets easily overwhelmed by noise and during transitions periods (e.g., from group to lunch, getting ready to leave, etc.). Maura will remain in the day program as long as they can handle her behavior, but then will require a different placement. Staff enjoy Maura and are willing to try and accommodate to her needs for as long as possible.

Occupational Therapy Evaluation

Maura has no deficits in sensation, vision, or hearing. It is felt that she might have some perceptual issues in body scheme and spatial orientation, but formalized testing hasn't been done. She was given the Allen's Cognitive Level test (ACL) and scored a 3.5. She is forgetful, requiring reminders and orientation to the daily schedule. She often gets to the center and asks for breakfast even though she has already had it at home. She insists that she hasn't, so the staff give her some toast and tea. She has poor problem-solving skills, but can perform automatic tasks well. She often repeats the same stories, and some other clients get annoyed at this and tell her to be quiet.

Maura has been lucky in that she has not had a lot of pain due to her AIDS. She does have poor endurance, tiring very easily during walks or exercise group. She takes a nap in the afternoon in one of the reclining chairs. Maura has difficulty identifying interests when doing the interest checklist. She likes loud rock music and watching TV, but that is all she can identify.

Maura comes to the day program clean and well-groomed. She says that her mother does her hair for her and takes good care of her.

Maura is unable to identify goals for herself. Staff have identified goals that include helping Maura during transitions, providing structure for her to help her function in the program, and giving staff guidance in how to deal with her confusion.

QUESTIONS

Goals/Treatment Plan

1. What are Maura's strengths and deficits?

2. Write a problem list for Maura.

3. What does the score on the ACL mean and how will it help you in your treatment planning?

4. Write long- and short-term goals for Maura.

5. What frame of reference will you use in working with Maura? What are the different frames of reference for working with individuals with cognitive deficits?

Safety/Precautions

6. What safety issues can you identify for Maura in the day program?

7. What might be some safety issues for her at home?

Self-Care/Work/Leisure

8. Maura's mother has told the staff that she has to dress Maura because she gets confused and doesn't dress properly (she might forget to put on her underwear or put on shorts in the winter). What can you suggest for techniques to assist her family in this area?

9. Maura's mother also tells the staff that Maura resents taking showers and gets very agitated when it is tried. What can you suggest to her to address this performance area?

10. Can you work on the problem discussed in Questions 8 and 9 in the day program? How?

11. You notice that when Maura eats lunch that she uses her hands instead of the utensils. How can you address this issue?

12. What types of craft projects do you think Maura would be able to do, and how would you grade and adapt these for her?

13. Maura enjoys the cooking and meal-planning group that occurs at the day program. This group involves the participants in making a complete lunch for the group, including shopping for the ingredients. Complete an activity analysis on this activity and then decide what parts of the activity, with or without adaptation, Maura could successfully do with minimal assistance.

14. Maura's parents say that weekends are tough because she just sits and watches TV all day. They would like to know if there are any activities, exercises, or anything else that they can have her do during the weekends. What do you suggest to them?

Equipment/Adaptations

15. What, if any, adaptive equipment would you give Maura for dressing and feeding? Why give her adaptive equipment for these activities? Why not?

16. How might you suggest to the staff that transition times be adapted for Maura so that she is better able to cope with them?

NOTES

Neuromusculoskeletal

17. What type of activities would you do with Maura to help with her endurance issues?

Cognition/Perception

18. List Maura's cognitive and perceptual issues and what impact they may have on her functioning at home and at the day program.

19. What types of group activities would be beneficial for Maura to attend that might address some of these issues?

20. Are there suggestions you would make to the staff that would help them deal with Maura's cognitive and perceptual issues?

21. Create an outline for an in-service to give to staff to address the impact of these cognitive and perceptual issues on Maura's daily functioning.

Psychosocial

22. Maura has been refusing to come to groups for about a week now, stating that she is going to die anyway, so she does not want to bother doing anything. What can you do to re-engage her in the OT groups?

23. Maura can be very disruptive during groups, especially with her inappropriate responses pointed at other people in the group. How would you handle this behavior in your OT groups?

Patient/Family Education

24. Maura's parents are wondering what the course of her disease will be so they can plan for the future and know whether they need to find alternative sources of care for her. What resources can you find to give to them?

Situations

25. Maura becomes agitated when a new person joins the day program. She attempts to push the woman when they are out on a group walk. How do you handle this, and what can be done to prevent it from happening again?

26. Maura refuses to get on the van to come to the program for the second day in a row. Her mother calls looking for advice and help. What do you tell her?

Discharge Planning

27. Since you are on the staff of the day program, Maura is not discharged from occupational therapy. How often would you update your plan of care for her and do re-evaluations on the ACL?

NOTES

Chapter 40

Nancy:
Depression

Nancy is a 56-year-old African-American female who attends a day hospital program 5 days a week. She has a diagnosis of depression. She came to the day program after a 2-week acute inpatient hospitalization for depression. She became quite despondent when her only son committed suicide. She blames herself for not recognizing that he was depressed and wanted to kill himself. Her son lived with her and worked full-time. She continued to function in her job as a computer programming specialist for several weeks after his death, but soon began to call in sick and eventually just did not show up. She <u>had</u> difficulty getting out of bed in the morning and finally stopped trying altogether. Her ex-husband grew concerned when he only got the answering machine for several days. He went over to her apartment, and she answered the door in her nightgown. The apartment had not been cleaned (Nancy is typically very neat) and there was no food in the refrigerator; there were frozen-food containers all over the kitchen. Nancy responded to his questions with one-word answers. He called her physician who recommended he take her to the emergency room. The psychiatric team did an assessment and decided that she required inpatient hospitalization. She was cooperative during her stay, but did not respond to conventional medication, so a series of electroconvulsive therapy (ECT) treatments were continued on an outpatient basis. The results of ECT were good, but she had some short-term memory loss. It was felt that she was not ready to return to her job and placement was sought in the day program for continued support and therapy. Nancy has a history of depression in her family. Her mother was hospitalized when Nancy was young for a "nervous breakdown" and her grandfather also had a history of mental illness, but Nancy does not know what his diagnosis was.

Nancy's goal is to return to work. She is expected to participate in the activities of the day program and the groups both she and the team select.

Occupational Therapy Evaluation

Nancy has no deficits in sensation, hearing, vision, or perception. She has some short-term memory loss from the ECT and appears confused at times, but these side effects should clear within a few weeks. She scored a 5 on the Allen's Cognitive Levels test. She is being driven to the day program by her ex-husband. She has a flat affect, speaks softly, and answers in one- or two-word responses. Nancy does not note many interests on the interest checklist, but when reviewed with her on a one-on-one basis, she is able to identify past interests in reading, cooking, traveling, and gardening. She notes that since her divorce 12 years ago, she spends most of her time at work. Since her boss is often in on the weekends, she goes in to help him. When she doesn't go in, she goes to the movies or shopping alone. She does not identify any close friends, stating "I didn't need them. I had my husband and son." She closely identifies with the role of caretaker and worker; however, she feels she must have been a terrible caretaker if the two people she cared for are not with her anymore.

She remains rather listless and is poorly motivated at the day program. She interacts minimally with the other clients, although there is another woman around her age who is also attending and she has tried to make friends with Nancy.

Nancy's goal is to return to her job. Her boss has promised that the job will be there as soon as she is ready to come back.

QUESTIONS

Goals/Treatment Plan

1. What do you see as Nancy's strengths and weaknesses?

2. What, if any, obstacles do you see in Nancy reaching her goal?

3. What are the long- and short-term goals for Nancy?

4. What frame of reference will you use in treatment with Nancy?

5. Using the Model of Human Occupation, how would you describe Nancy's volitional and habituation subsystems?

Safety/Precautions

6. What precautions do you need to take with Nancy in the day program?

Self-Care/Work/Leisure

7. What types of skills do you feel Nancy has to work on in order to be able to return to work?

8. What activities can you do to address her work skills?

9. What types of groups do you think Nancy would benefit from in the day program?

10. How can you help Nancy re-engage in some of her expressed interests?

Equipment/Adaptations

11. How would you address assisting Nancy in developing a balanced routine of work and leisure activities?

Cognition/Perception

12. What methods can you use to teach Nancy to compensate for her short-term memory loss from ECT?

13. How can you ensure that Nancy uses these techniques outside of the day program?

Psychosocial

14. What possible outside supports can you identify for Nancy?

15. Nancy does not interact with other clients at the day program. Why do you think she may not interact with others?

16. What activities can you suggest that would help Nancy interact with others in the program? Who might be a good individual to try and connect Nancy with?

17. Nancy does not show motivation to initiate activities or to go to groups on her own. She always needs reminders and coaxing to attend. What can you do to improve her motivation and initiation?

NOTES

Patient/Family Education

18. Please find some educational materials for Nancy about depression.

19. What do you feel is important for Nancy to know about depression? Why do you think this information is important?

Situations

20. Nancy comes to group one day and shares that an old friend has contacted her and wants to get together. This friend doesn't know about Nancy's psychiatric illness. She is nervous about getting together. How would you advise her?

Discharge Planning

21. Nancy is to be discharged from the day program with a plan to return to work part-time and a goal of full-time work within a few months. What recommendations can you make to Nancy to ensure that she spends her non-working time productively?

NOTES

INDEX

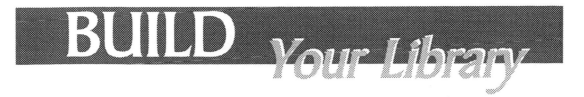

BUILD *Your Library*

This book and many others on numerous different topics are available from SLACK Incorporated. For further information or a copy of our latest catalog, please contact us at:

Professional Book Division
SLACK Incorporated
6900 Grove Road
Thorofare, NJ 08086 USA
Telephone: 1-856-848-1000
1-800-257-8290
Fax: 1-856-853-5991
E-mail: orders@slackinc.com
www.slackbooks.com

We accept most major credit cards and checks or money orders in US dollars drawn on a US bank. Most orders are shipped within 72 hours.

Contact us for information on recent releases, forthcoming titles, and bestsellers. If you have a comment about this title or see a need for a new book, direct your correspondence to the Editorial Director at the above address.

Thank you for your interest and we hope you found this work beneficial.